CONTENTS

INTRODUCTION

The Ninja® Foodi™ Digital Air Fryer Oven is built on the raving reviews of the other Ninja® Foodi™ kitchen appliances. The original food chopper has been a huge success with over 4.5 stars and almost 2,000 reviews on Amazon. This new oven is the same concept but scaled up to meet the needs of crispy air fryer style cooking.

One of the major draws for this option. Is its capacity of 3 ⅓ quarts. It's much bigger than its competitors, like the VonShef Digital Air Fryer (2 quarts) or other larger traditional countertop fryers (4–8 quarts). Bigger volume means that you can make more food at once, more servings of a single meal with ease, and less time spent prepping and cooking food. It's great for a lot of different meals that require the use of less oil.

The Ninja Foodi Digital Air Fry Oven is easy to use and includes all the important features you need.

It has a capacity of 3 ⅓ quarts with a 360°F heating element and rotisserie mechanism (also known as convection) for even heat distribution throughout your food. It can bake, grill, roast, and air fry foods at once! No more having to cook multiple separately! The unit is also super easy to clean and maintain thanks to its removable drip tray.

The countertop model comes with an LCD display and digital timer. The display shows the temperature, time, and menu programming options. You can also set a countdown timer to let you know when the food is done cooking.

With the new Ninja Foodi Digital Air Fry Oven, you can make delicious homemade foods without worrying about wasting food or excess oil. Most meals take less than 10 minutes from start to finish! This is perfect for people with busy lifestyles that don't have the time to spend in the kitchen or at home all day every day! Get started right away with this easy-to-use unit that has all the features you need right out of the box.

We are going to take an in-depth look at the Ninja Foodi Digital Air Fry Oven. Its features and uses will help you easily find the perfect recipes for your individual lifestyle and cooking needs.

The Ninja Foodi Digital Air Fry Oven Cookbook is a great addition to any home kitchen! This is a great addition to your kitchen if you are getting started with air frying because it has so many different recipes that will allow you to get started in a number of different ways. This Cookbook comes fully loaded with some of the best recipes out there that you can make with the handy and user-friendly air fryer.

This is a great addition for anyone who is just getting into air frying. They can easily find recipes that will help them continue learning and experimenting with their new appliance. The unit comes with plenty of different recipes that will help you get started in creating some delicious homemade meals right away!

The type of air fryer also comes with plenty of accessories, including cooking racks and tongs, which make cleaning up easy after use.

Let yourself be inspired by this complete and straightforward cookbook. Thanks to the number of recipes contained and their simplicity, you can easily alternate these delicacies to get 1000 days of simple and creative cuisine.

Whether you are a beginner or an expert, this cookbook will give you the possibility to satisfy your palate, along with that of your friends and family, without ever getting bored, thanks to 1000 days of alternatives.

CHAPTER 1: THE NINJA FOODI DIGITAL AIR FRY OVEN BASICS

What is the Ninja Foodi Digital Air Fryer?

The Ninja Foodi Air Fry is the ultimate meal-making machine. It is a convection oven with smart-programmed features that lets you cook a complete dish meal using just one kitchen device. This elegant and revolutionary kitchen appliance allows you to cook with any of its 8 cooking modes, even when you're not endowed with culinary skill.

Functionalities

- **Air Fry:** It allows air frying without or less oil added.
- **Air Roast:** It produces a perfectly browned, crispy, and evenly-cooked dishes, like a full-sized sheet pan with roasted vegetables.
- **Air Broil:** It allows you to broil fish and meat and brown casserole tops evenly.
- **Bake:** It allows you to conveniently bake pastries, desserts, and snacks.
- **Dehydrate:** It is useful for dehydrating meat, vegetables, and fruits.
- **Keep Warm:** It can keep your food warm up to 2 hours.
- **Toast:** It allows you to toast up to 9 bread slices simultaneously with "Light," "Dark," and "Brown" options.
- **Bagel:** You can perfectly toast up to 9 bagel halves when placed cut-side up on the wire rack.

Advantages of Using Ninja Digital Air Fry Oven
Made of High-Quality Material

The oven is made of stainless steel with rounded edges and coated with a superb finishing that makes it look elegant and classy. This material gives the air fryer durability and strength. With careful use, the oven could last for years.

Save Enough Counter Space

The Air Fry Oven takes up 50% less space in your countertop or cabinet, as you can have the option to flip it up and store it. It has an adjustable flip function that allows you to keep the oven in both vertical and horizontal positions on your counter or kitchen shelf—depending on available space. However, when you are ready to store it while not in use, simply flip it up and it can stand in a vertical position, leaving more space (about 50%) on your shelf for your other kitchen appliance.

Another thing that makes this Air Fry Oven a real space saver is the fact that you won't need toasters, as the Ninja Foodie Digital Air Fry Oven is also a useful toaster that gives you two options for toasting bread slices and bagel. Simply press the "Toast" button for bread or the "Bagel" button for toasting a bagel.

You can adjust the temperature and time for toasts when you press the "Darkness" button and "Slices" button. These functions can provide you with a crispy dark brown or soft light brown toast depending on what you desire.

Speed Cooking

It can Cook 60% faster compared to when you're using a traditional oven with an air roast. You can preheat the oven in 60 seconds and have a full meal in as little as 20 minutes.

Beautiful Design

- Easy to navigate as digital controls are basic and simple
- Soundless
- Retain
- An excellent toaster and best for sheet pans
- An even toast on both light and medium settings
- Excellent for sheet pan dinner

Easy to Clean

It would be easy to clean this cooking appliance as the entire meal is prepared on a sheet pan, making cleaning a quick and easy job to do. The Ninja Foodi Digital Air Fry Oven is also equipped with a crumb tray that gets hold of falling debris and residues from the air fryer. It also protects the bottom of the oven from spilling. You can also easily get access to the back panel for deep cleaning, as the oven is provided with a large opening at the back that enables you to clean the entire surface properly. Just use soap and a damp towel when cleaning.

Easy to Understand Manual

The Ninja Foodi Digital Air Fry Oven comes with an instructional manual that contains detailed instructions, recipes, and charts to guide you in air frying and dehydrating. It also guides you on how to make your sheet pan meal even though there is no guide for baking, air broiling, and air roasting.

The oven preheats automatically for one minute and unlike other nosy air fryers, Ninja Foodi Digital Air Fry Oven is almost soundless. It is easy to check on the progress of the dish you're cooking with its LED light on.

It is also easy to clean up, as the sheet pan and the air fry basket are dishwasher-friendly, although you must not touch it right after cooking as the oven remains too hot. Allow the oven to cool down before cleaning it up to avoid getting your skin burnt.

For those who intend to buy an oven toaster and an air fryer, the Ninja Foodi Digital Air Fry Oven is worth a try.

Features of Ninja Foodi Digital Air Fry Oven

Air Fry Basket

The flat air fry basket accommodates more food compared to the rounded one currently available in most air fryer models. You can evenly spread your food out to produce an even distribution of hot air, resulting in well-browned crisp air fried dishes.

Depending on your recipe, the basket can hold up to 4 lb. of food, but to ensure even cooking, follow the directions in your recipe. It is also non-stick, so it is not necessary to spray it with cooking oil to prevent it from sticking.

Sheet Pan

The Ninja Foodi Digital Air Fry Oven comes with a sheet pan that sits just below the air fry basket, catching any falling crumbs or dripping grease from the food you are cooking. There is neither grove nor space to allow the pan to be moved without moving the air fryer basket, and vice versa. So when removing the hot air fryer basket while cooking, you need to keep in mind removing it together with the pan to avoid accidentally having it landed on your foot.

Side Blower

The Ninja Foodi Digital Air Fry Oven blows in the air coming from the sides as opposed to the usual top-down approach use by most air fryers. When the food is evenly spread on the air fryer basket, the hot air coming in from the sides can produce a crispier result and a more even browning.

The Control Panel

You would not find it difficult to navigate through your cooking experiences as the digital control panel on the Ninja Foodie Digital Air Fry Oven is easy to read and understand. The interface is fairly intuitive to set and is centered on a knob or dial that you can turn to set the cooking time and temperature for each function. It also allows you to select the number of slices and doneness. The Ninja Foodie Digital Air Fry Oven has a LED screen just above the control panel that displays the temperature in "F" as well as the cooking time in minutes and hours. If the oven is preheating, you will see "Pre" displayed on the screen, or "Hot" if it needs a little cooling. Once it has cooled enough, the display will show "Flip," which means that the Air Fry Oven can now be flipped and ready to be stored.

Ninja Digital Air Fry Oven Smart Settings

It is very easy to follow as each button in the control signifies every function. In addition to air frying, the oven works on multiple functions traditionally covered by ovens and toasters respectively, including baking and broiling. It also includes a dehydrator if you wish to dehydrator fruits and meats.

Functions and modes are right below the LED panel. It has a multifunctional dial that serves as the selector for the preferred function and also starts/pauses the oven. The "Temperature" and "Time" buttons are for adjusting the cooking temperature and time. There is also an adjustment for the darkness level and the number of slices for the "Toast" mode. Take notice that the "Bagel" and "Toast" modes don't display time and temperature; instead, they show the darkness level and the number of slices. To easily change from one mode to another, simply rotate the selector dial. The current mode is indicated by the blue light.

The "ON" and "OFF" power buttons can be found close to the control panel.

Air Fry:

- **Heat Source/Airflow:** High heat from top and bottom
- **Desired Result or Effect:** Quick and extra-crispy effect with little or no oil
- **Requirement:** An air fryer with or without sheet pan

- **Best for:** French fries (freshly cut or frozen), chicken wings, and vegetables

Air Roast:
- **Heat Source/Airflow:** Even heat from top and bottom
- **Desired Result or Effect:** A dish that is crispy on the outside but juicy inside
- **Requirement:** A sheet pan
- **Best for:** Sheet pan meals, whole meat, and vegetables

Air Broil:
- **Heat Source/Airflow:** High heat from top
- **Desired Result or Effect:** Top-down heat for a crispy effect
- **Best for:** Fish, nachos, steak, and for finishing casseroles
- **Requirement:** A sheet pan

Bake:
- **Heat Source/Airflow:** High, even heat from top and bottom
- **Desired Result or Effect:** Overall even cooking with light-browning effect
- **Best for:** Cookies, cakes, and frozen pizza
- **Requirement:** Use a sheet pan

Toast:
- **Heat Source/Airflow:** Even heat from top and bottom
- **Desired Result or Effect:** Quick even browning effect on both sides
- **Best for:** English muffins, bread, and frozen waffles
- **Requirement:** Use a wire rack

Bagel:
- **Heat Source/Airflow:** Slightly lower heat from the top than the bottom
- **Desired Result or Effect:** Quick, even browning
- **Best for:** Bagels and artisan bread
- **Requirement:** A wire rack

Dehydrate:
- **Heat Source/Airflow:** Low Heat
- **Desired Result or Effect:** Removed moisture for jerky and dried fruits
- **Best for:** Jerky and dried fruits
- **Requirement:** The air fryer basket with or without sheet pan

Dehydrating
When you want to make use of the dehydration feature of the Ninja Foodi Digital Air Fry, here are some kitchen tips to make things easier and better.

To lessen dehydrating time and save on energy, you need to slice fruits and vegetables to a thin size. It would be easier to use a mandolin slicer to produce uniformed cuts.

Some fruits oxidize when cut. Soak them in water mixed with squeezed lemon extract for 5 minutes. This will prevent discoloration and help them retain their color while undergoing the process of dehydration.

Before adding fruits and veggies to your Air Fry Oven to dehydrate, pat them dry with paper towels. This will help decrease the time needed to dehydrate the fruits or veggies.

Lay each piece of the food flat on the air fry basket without stacking them or overlapping them with each other so that the circulating hot air can easily reach them.

On average, fruits and vegetables require low heat (135ºF) and takes about 6–8 hours to dehydrate. When dehydrating fresh food, check every 6 hours to monitor the degree of doneness and prevent the food from getting burnt.

You can maximize the longevity of dehydrated food by storing them at room temperature in an air-tight container for up to two weeks. If you plan to dehydrate fish and meat, it is recommended that you roast them at 330ºF for about 1 minute as a final step to completely pasteurize them. For jerky, it gets crispier when you dehydrate them longer.

Digital Time and Temperature Setting

The digital display makes it easy to set your cooking time and temperature based on your recipe. To set cooking time, simply press the "Time" button and rotate the dial to the desired time. To set the cooking temperature, set the "Temp" button and rotate the dial to set it to the desired temperature. To start cooking, press on the dial.

When setting, the temperature range can vary depending on the function.
- For air frying, the temperature range can be between 250–450ºF.
- For air roasting, the temperature range can be between 250–450ºF.
- For air broiling, the temperature range can be between 350–450ºF (high).
- For baking, the temperature range can be between 250–400ºF.
- For toasting, the temperature can be up to 450ºF.
- For dehydrating, the temperature range can be between 105–195ºF.
- For warming food previously cooked, the temperature can be up to 165ºF.

When setting the cooking time, the time increments can vary also depending on the preferred function.
- For air frying, the time increment is 1 min–1 hour.
- For air roasting, the time increment is 1 min–2 hours.
- For air broiling, the time increment is 30 sec–30 min.
- For air baking, the time increment is 1 min–2 hours.
- For toasting, the time increment is 30 sec–10 min, depending on the "Darkness" and "Slice" settings.
- For dehydrating, the time increment is 30 min–12 hours.
- For keeping food warm, the time increment is 5 min–2 hours.

Taking Care of Your Air Fryer

Regular cleaning is essential to ensure that your Ninja Foodi Digital Air Fry Oven can last long, regular cleaning is essential. We have here two guides to cleaning your revolutionary kitchen device.

For Everyday Cleaning

After each use, unplug your Ninja Foodi Digital Air Fry Oven from the wall outlet. But before cleaning, make sure that it has cooled off as the oven can be very hot and can burn your skin. You will see the "HOT" sign in red that will tell you that the cooling is still in progress. Once it has completely cooled down, the "HOT" sign will disappear, which means that it is now ready for cleaning and you can now unplug the oven to cut the power supply. You can then start taking out all the removable parts including the wire rack, sheet pan, air fryer basket, and crumb tray.

Slide out the crumb tray and empty it of crumbs and other burnt residues that have fallen off from the air fryer basket.

Clean the inside of the cooking chamber and the control panel by wiping it with a clean, damp cloth. This would leave your Ninja Foodi Digital Air Fry Oven sparkling clean and ready for the next use.

For Deep Cleaning

Make sure that you have unplugged your Ninja Foodi Digital Air Fry Oven from the wall outlet or socket and have left it to cool down.

Start removing all accessories from your Air Fry Oven, including the crumb tray. Wash each accessory separately. Note that all parts of the Ninja Foodi Digital Air Fry Oven are dishwasher-friendly.

Flip the oven up into the storage position and press the "Push" button to release the back door. This will provide you access to the interior of the Air Fry Oven.

Use warm, soapy water and a soft cloth to wash the interior side of the Air Fry Oven. Avoid using abrasive cleansers, chemical-based cleaners, and scrubbing brushes to clean, for it can damage the unit. Never submerge the main unit either in the dishwasher, in water, or any liquid. Only the removable parts such as the sheet pan, rack, and air fryer basket are dishwasher-friendly.

Do not forget to thoroughly dry all parts before placing them back in the oven for future use.

To flip the air fryer up, hold the handle under the lid and try pushing its front upward. Then pull the base of the oven and it will likewise come out like the lid. Also, wipe the base with a damp cloth and allow complete drying for the base before closing it.

CHAPTER 2: BREAKFAST

Delicious Breakfast Soufflé

Preparation Time: 5 minutes
Cooking Time: 15 minutes
Servings: 4
Ingredients:

- 6 eggs
- ⅓ cup milk
- ½ cup shredded mozzarella cheese
- 1 tbsp. freshly chopped parsley
- ½ cup chopped ham
- 1 tsp. salt
- 1 tsp. black pepper
- ½ tsp. garlic powder
- Cooking spray

Directions:

1. Grease 4 ramekins with a non-stick cooking spray. Preheat your Air Fry Oven to 350ºF.
2. Using a large bowl, add and stir all the ingredients until they are mixed properly.
3. Pour the egg mixture into the greased ramekins and place it inside your Air Fry Oven.
4. Cook it inside your air fryer for 8 minutes. Then carefully remove the soufflé from your air fryer and allow it to cool off.
5. Serve and enjoy!

Nutrition:

- Calories: 195
- Fats: 15 g
- Carbs: 6 g
- Protein: 9 g

Yummy Breakfast Italian Frittata

Preparation Time: 5 minutes
Cooking Time: 10 minutes
Servings: 6
Ingredients:

- 6 eggs
- ⅓ cup milk
- 4-oz. chopped Italian sausage
- 3 cups stemmed and roughly chopped kale
- 1 red seeded and chopped bell pepper
- ½ cup a grated feta cheese
- 1 chopped zucchini
- 1 tbsp. freshly chopped basil
- 1 tsp. garlic powder
- 1 tsp. onion powder
- 1 tsp. salt
- 1 tsp. black pepper

Directions:

1. Preheat your Air Fry Oven to 360°F.
2. Grease the air fryer pan with a non-stick cooking spray.
3. Add the Italian sausage to the pan and cook it inside your Air Fry Oven for 5 minutes.
4. While doing that, add and stir in the remaining ingredients until they mix properly.
5. Add the egg mixture to the pan and allow it to cook inside your Air Fry Oven for 5 minutes.
6. Then carefully remove the pan and allow it to cool off until it gets chill enough to serve.
7. Serve and enjoy!

Nutrition:

- Calories: 225
- Fats: 14 g
- Carbs: 4.5 g
- Protein: 20 g

Savory Cheese and Bacon Muffins

Preparation Time: 5 minutes
Cooking Time: 17 minutes
Servings: 4
Ingredients:

- 1 ½ cup all-purpose flour
- 2 tsp. baking powder
- ½ cup milk
- 2 eggs
- 1 tbsp. freshly chopped parsley
- 4 cooked and chopped bacon slices
- 1 thinly chopped onion
- ½ cup shredded cheddar cheese
- ½ tsp. onion powder
- 1 tsp. salt
- 1 tsp. black pepper

Directions:

1. Turn on your Air Fry Oven and let it heat up to 360ºF.

2. In a large bowl, add and stir all the ingredients until they mix properly.

3. Then grease the muffin cups with a non-stick cooking spray or line it with parchment paper. The pour the batter proportionally into each muffin cup.

4. Place it inside your Air Fry Oven and bake it for 15 minutes.

5. Then carefully remove it from your Air Fry Oven and allow it to chill.

6. Serve and enjoy!

Nutrition:
- Calories: 180
- Fats: 18 g
- Carbs: 16 g
- Protein: 15 g

Best Air-Fried English Breakfast

Preparation Time: 5 minutes
Cooking Time: 20 minutes
Servings: 4
Ingredients:
- 8 sausages
- 8 bacon slices
- 4 eggs
- 1 (16-oz.) can baked beans
- 8 slices of toast

Directions:
1. Add the sausages and bacon slices to your air fryer and cook them for 10 minutes at a 320°F.

2. In a ramekin or heat-resistant bowl, add the baked beans, place another ramekin, and add the eggs and whisk.

3. Increase the temperature to 290°F.

4. Place it inside your air fryer and cook it for an additional 10 minutes, or until everything is done.

5. Serve and enjoy!

Nutrition:
- Calories: 850
- Fats: 40 g
- Carbs: 20 g
- Protein: 48 g

Sausage and Egg Breakfast Burrito

Preparation Time: 5 minutes
Cooking Time: 30 minutes
Servings: 6

Ingredients:
- 6 eggs
- Salt
- Pepper
- Cooking oil
- ½ cup chopped red bell pepper
- ½ cup chopped green bell pepper
- 8 oz. ground chicken sausage
- ½ cup salsa
- 6 medium (8-inch) flour tortillas
- ½ cup shredded Cheddar cheese

Directions:
1. In a medium bowl, whisk the eggs, and add salt and pepper to taste.

2. Place a skillet in the air fryer on medium-high heat. Spray with cooking oil. Add the egg and scramble them for 2–3 minutes, until the eggs are fluffy. Remove the eggs from the skillet and set aside.

3. If needed, spray the skillet with more oil. Add the chopped red and green bell peppers. Cook for 2–3 minutes, or until the peppers are soft.

4. Add the ground sausage to the skillet. Break the sausage into smaller pieces using a spatula or spoon. Then cook for 3–4 minutes, or until the sausage is brown.

5. Add the salsa and scrambled eggs. Stir to combine. Remove the skillet from heat.

6. Spoon the mixture evenly onto the tortillas.

7. To form the burritos, fold the sides of each tortilla toward the middle and then roll up from the bottom. You can secure each burrito with a toothpick. Alternatively, you can moisten the outside edge of the tortilla with a small amount of water. I prefer to use a cooking brush, but you can also dab with your fingers.

8. Spray the burritos with cooking oil and place them in the Air Fry Oven. Do not stack. Cook the burritos in batches if they do not all fit in the basket. Cook for 8 minutes

9. Open the Air Fry Oven and flip the burritos. Heat it for an additional 2 minutes or until crisp.

10. If necessary, repeat steps 8 and 9 for the remaining burritos.

11. Sprinkle the Cheddar cheese over the burritos. Cool before serving.

Nutrition:
- Calories: 236 Fats: 13 g

- Carbs: 16 g Protein: 15 g

French Toast Sticks

Preparation Time: 5 minutes
Cooking Time: 15 minutes
Servings: 12
Ingredients:

- 4 slices Texas toast (or any thick bread, such as challah)
- 1 tbsp. butter
- 1 egg
- 1 tsp. stevia
- 1 tsp. ground cinnamon
- ¼ cup milk
- 1 tsp. vanilla extract
- Cooking oil

Directions:

1. Cut each bread slice into 3 pieces (for 12 sticks total).
2. Place the butter in a small, microwave-safe bowl. Heat for 15 seconds or until the butter has melted.
3. Remove the bowl from the microwave. Add the egg, stevia, cinnamon, milk, and vanilla extract. Whisk until fully combined.
4. Spray the air fry basket with cooking oil.
5. Dredge each of the bread sticks in the egg mixture.
6. Place the French toast sticks in the Air Fry Oven—it is okay to stack them. Spray the French toast sticks with cooking oil. Cook for 8 minutes
7. Open the Air Fry Oven and flip each of the French toast sticks. Cook for an additional 4 minutes or until the French toast sticks are crisp.
8. Cool before serving.

Nutrition:

- Calories: 52
- Fats: 2 g
- Carbs: 7 g
- Protein: 2 g

Home-Fried Potatoes

Preparation Time: 5 minutes
Cooking Time: 25 minutes
Servings: 4
Ingredients:

- 3 large russet potatoes
- 1 tbsp. canola oil
- 1 tbsp. extra-virgin olive oil
- 1 tsp. paprika
- Salt
- Pepper
- 1 cup chopped onion
- 1 cup chopped red bell pepper
- 1 cup chopped green bell pepper

Directions:

1. Cut the potatoes into ½-inch cubes. Place the potatoes in a large bowl of cold water and allow them to soak for at least 30 minutes, preferably an hour.
2. Dry out the potatoes and wipe thoroughly with paper towels. Then return them to the empty bowl.
3. Add the canola and olive oils, paprika, and salt and pepper to flavor. Toss to fully coat the potatoes.
4. Transfer the potatoes to the Air Fry Oven. Cook for 20 minutes, shaking the air fryer basket every 5 minutes (a total of 4 times).
5. Place the onion and red and green bell peppers in the air fry basket. Fry for an additional 3–4 minutes, or until the potatoes are cooked through and the peppers are soft.
6. Cool before serving.

Nutrition:

- Calories: 279
- Fats: 8 g
- Carbs: 50 g
- Protein: 6 g

Homemade Cherry Breakfast Tarts

Preparation Time: 15 minutes
Cooking Time: 20 minutes
Servings: 6
Ingredients:
For the Tarts:

- 2 refrigerated piecrusts
- ⅓ cup cherry preserves
- 1 tsp. cornstarch
- Cooking oil

For the Frosting:

- ½ cup vanilla yogurt
- 1 oz. cream cheese
- 1 tsp. stevia

- 1 tsp. Rainbow sprinkles

Directions:

1. To make the tarts, Place the piecrusts on a flat surface. Then cut each piecrust with a pizza cutter, for 6 in total. (I discard the unused dough left from slicing the edges).

2. In a small bowl, combine the preserves and cornstarch. Mix well.

3. Scoop 1 tbsp. of the preserve mixture onto the top half of each piece of piecrust.

4. Fold the bottom of each piece up to close the tart. Press along the edges of each tart to seal them using the back of a fork.

5. Sprinkle the breakfast tarts with cooking oil and place them in the Air Fry Oven. I do not recommend piling the breakfast tarts because they will stick together if piled, so you may need to prepare them in two batches. Cook for 10 minutes.

6. Allow the breakfast tarts to cool fully before removing them from the Air Fry Oven.

7. If needed, repeat steps 5 and 6 for the remaining breakfast tarts.

8. To make the frosting, mix well the yogurt, cream cheese, and stevia in a small bowl.

9. Spread the breakfast tarts with frosting, top with sprinkles, and serve.

Nutrition:
- Calories: 119
- Fats: 4 g
- Carbs: 19 g
- Protein: 2 g

Sausage and Cream Cheese Biscuits

Preparation Time: 5 minutes
Cooking Time: 15 minutes
Serving: 5
Ingredients:
- 12 oz. chicken breakfast sausage
- 1 (6-oz.) can biscuits
- ⅛ cup cream cheese

Direction:

1. Form 5 sausage patties out of the sausages.

2. Place the sausage patties in the Air Fry Oven and cook for 5 minutes

3. Open the air fryer, flip the patties, and cook for an additional 5 minutes.

4. Remove the cooked sausages from the air fryer.

5. Form 5 biscuits out of the biscuit dough.

6. Place the biscuits in the air fryer and cook for 3 minutes.

7. Open the Air Fry Oven, flip the biscuits, and cook for an additional 2 minutes.

8. Remove the cooked biscuits from the air fryer.

9. Split each biscuit in half. Spread 1 tsp. of cream cheese onto the bottom of each biscuit. Top with a sausage patty and the other half of the biscuit. Serve.

Nutrition:
- Calories: 24 g
- Fats: 13 g
- Carbs: 20 g
- Protein: 9 g

Fried Chicken and Waffles

Preparation Time: 10 minutes
Cooking Time: 30 minutes
Servings: 4
Ingredients:
- 8 whole chicken wings
- 1 tsp. garlic powder
- Chicken seasoning or rub
- Pepper
- ½ cup all-purpose flour
- Cooking oil
- 8 frozen waffles
- Maple syrup (optional)

Directions:

1. In a medium bowl, spice the chicken with garlic powder, chicken seasoning, and pepper to flavor.

2. Put the chicken in a sealable plastic bag and add the flour. Shake to thoroughly coat the chicken.

3. Spray the air fry basket with cooking oil.

4. With the use of tongs, transfer the chicken from the bag to the air fryer. Pile the chickens on top of each other. Sprinkle them with cooking oil. Heat for five minutes

5. Unlock the air fryer and shake the basket. Proceed to cook the chicken. Keep shaking every 5 minutes until 20 minutes has passed, or until the chicken is completely cooked.

6. Take out the cooked chicken from the air fryer and set it aside.

7. Wash the basket with warm water. Then transfer them back to the air fryer.

8. Lower the temperature of the Air Fry Oven to 370ºF.

9. Put the frozen waffles in the Air Fry Oven, without piling them. Depending on how big your air fryer is, you may need to cook the waffles in batches. Sprinkle the waffles with cooking oil. Cook for 6 minutes.

10. If necessary, take out the cooked waffles from the Air Fry Oven, then repeat step 9 for the leftover waffles.

11. Serve the waffles with the chicken and a bit of maple syrup if desired.

Nutrition:
- Calories: 461
- Fats: 22 g
- Carbs: 45 g
- Protein: 28 g

Cheesy Tater Tot Breakfast Bake

Preparation Time: 5 minutes
Cooking Time: 20 minutes
Servings: 4
Ingredients:
- 4 eggs
- 1 cup milk
- 1 tsp. onion powder
- Salt
- Pepper
- Cooking oil
- 12 oz. ground chicken sausage
- 1-lb. frozen tater tots
- ¾ cup shredded Cheddar cheese

Directions:
1. Whisk the eggs in medium bowls. Add the milk, onion powder, and salt and pepper to taste. Stir to combine.

2. Spray a skillet with cooking oil and place it over medium-high heat. Add the ground sausage. Using a spatula or spoon, cut the sausage into smaller pieces. Cook for 3–4 minutes, or until the sausage is brown. Remove from heat and set aside.

3. Spray a barrel pan with cooking oil. Make sure to oil the bottom and sides of the pan.

4. Place the tater tots in the barrel pan. Cook for 6 minutes in the Air Fry Oven.

5. Open the Air Fry Oven and shake the pan, then add the egg mixture and cooked sausage. Cook for an additional 6 minutes. Open the Air Fry Oven and sprinkle the cheese over the tater tot bake. Cook for an additional 2–3 minutes

6. Cool before serving.

Nutrition:
- Calories: 518
- Fats: 30 g
- Carbs: 31 g
- Protein: 30 g

Breakfast Scramble Casserole

Preparation Time: 20 minutes
Cooking Time: 10 minutes
Servings: 4
Ingredients:
- 6 slices bacon
- 6 eggs
- Salt
- Pepper
- Cooking oil
- ½ cup chopped red bell pepper
- ½ cup chopped green bell pepper
- ½ cup chopped onion
- ¾ cup shredded Cheddar cheese

Directions:
1. In a pan over medium-high heat, cook the bacon for 5–7 minutes, flipping until evenly crisp. Dry out on paper towels, crumble the bacon, and set aside. In a medium bowl, whisk the eggs. Add salt and pepper to taste.

2. Spray a barrel pan with cooking oil, especially the bottom and sides of the pan. Add the beaten eggs, crumbled bacon, red bell pepper, green bell pepper, and onion to the pan. Place the pan in the Air Fry Oven. Cook for 6 minutes Open the air fryer and sprinkle the cheese over the casserole. Cook for an additional 2 minutes. Cool before serving.

Nutrition:
- Calories: 348
- Fats: 26 g
- Carbs: 4 g
- Protein: 25 g

Breakfast Grilled Ham and Cheese

Preparation Time: 5 minutes
Cooking Time: 10 minutes
Servings: 2
Ingredients:

- 1 tsp. butter
- 4 slices bread
- 4 slices smoked country ham
- 4 slices Cheddar cheese
- 4 thick slices tomato

Directions:

1. Spread ½ tsp. of butter onto one side of 2 bread slices. Each sandwich will have 1 bread slice with butter and 1 slice without.
2. Assemble each sandwich by layering 2 ham slices, 2 cheese slices, and 2 tomato slices on the unbuttered bread pieces. Top with the other bread slices buttered-side up.
3. Place the sandwiches in the air fryer buttered-side down. Cook for 4 minutes
4. Open the air fryer, flip the grilled cheese sandwiches, and cook for an additional 4 minutes
5. Cool before serving. Cut each sandwich in half and enjoy.

Nutrition:

- Calories: 525
- Fats: 25 g
- Carbs: 34 g
- Protein: 41 g

Classic Hash Browns

Preparation Time: 15 minutes
Cooking Time: 20 minutes
Servings: 4
Ingredients:

- 4 russet potatoes
- 1 tsp. paprika
- Salt
- Pepper
- Cooking oil

Directions:

1. Peel the potatoes using a vegetable peeler. Shred the potatoes with a cheese grater. If your grater has differently sized holes, use the area of the tool with the largest holes.
2. Put the shredded potatoes in a large bowl of cold water. Let sit for 5 minutes Cold water helps remove excess starch from the potatoes. Stir to help dissolve the starch.
3. Dry out the potatoes with paper towels or napkins. Make sure the potatoes are completely dry.
4. Season the potatoes with paprika and salt and pepper to taste.
5. Spray the potatoes with cooking oil and transfer them to the Air Fry Oven. Cook for 20 minutes and shake the basket every 5 minutes (a total of 4 times).
6. Cool before serving.

Nutrition:

- Calories: 150
- Sodium: 52 mg
- Carbs: 34 g
- Fiber: 5 g
- Protein: 4 g

Canadian Bacon and Cheese English Muffins

Preparation Time: 5 minutes
Cooking Time: 10 minutes
Servings: 4
Ingredients:

- 4 English muffins
- 8 slices Canadian bacon
- 4 slices cheese
- Cooking oil

Directions:

1. Split each English muffin. Assemble the breakfast sandwiches by layering 2 Canadian bacon slices and 1 cheese slice into each English muffin bottom. Put the other half on top of the English muffin. Place the sandwiches in the Air Fry Oven. Spray the top of each with cooking oil. Cook for 4 minutes.
2. Open the Air Fry Oven and flip the sandwiches. Cook for an additional 4 minutes.
3. Cool before serving.

Nutrition:

- Calories: 333
- Fats: 14 g
- Carbs: 27 g
- Protein: 24 g

Radish Hash Browns

Preparation Time: 10 minutes

17

Cooking Time: 13 minutes

Servings: 4

Ingredients:

- 1 lb. radishes, washed and cut off roots
- 1 tbsp. olive oil
- ½ tsp. paprika
- ½ tsp. onion powder
- ½ tsp. garlic powder
- 1 medium onion
- ¼ tsp. pepper
- ¾ tsp. sea salt

Directions:

1. Slice the onion and radishes using a mandolin slicer.
2. Add the sliced onion and radishes to a large mixing bowl and toss with olive oil.
3. Transfer the onion and radish slices in an air fryer basket and cook at 360ºF for 8 minutes. Shake the basket twice.
4. Return the onion and radish slices to the mixing bowl and toss with seasonings.
5. Again, cook onion and radish slices in the air fry basket for 5 minutes at 400ºF. Shake the basket halfway through.
6. Serve and enjoy.

Nutrition:

- Calories: 62
- Fats: 3.7 g
- Carbs: 7.1 g
- Protein: 1.2 g

Vegetable Egg Cups

Preparation Time: 10 minutes

Cooking Time: 20 minutes

Servings: 4

Ingredients:

- 4 eggs
- 1 tbsp. cilantro, chopped
- 4 tbsp. half and half
- 1 cup cheddar cheese, shredded
- 1 cup vegetables, diced
- Pepper
- Salt

Directions:

1. Sprinkle 4 ramekins with cooking spray and set aside.
2. In a mixing bowl, whisk the eggs with cilantro, half and half, vegetables, ½ cup cheese, pepper, and salt.
3. Pour the egg mixture into the 4 ramekins.
4. Place ramekins in air fry basket and cook at 300ºF for 12 minutes.
5. Top with the remaining ½ cup of cheese and cook for 2 minutes more at 400ºF.
6. Serve and enjoy.

Nutrition:

- Calories: 194
- Fats: 11.5 g
- Carbs: 6 g
- Protein: 13 g

Spinach Frittata

Preparation Time: 5 minutes

Cooking Time: 8 minutes

Servings: 1

Ingredients:

- 3 eggs
- 1 cup spinach, chopped
- 1 small onion, minced
- 2 tbsp. mozzarella cheese, grated
- Pepper
- Salt

Directions:

1. Preheat the Air Fry Oven to 350ºF, and spray the sheet pan with cooking spray.
2. In a bowl, whisk the eggs with the remaining ingredients until well combined.
3. Pour the egg mixture into the prepared pan and place the pan in the air fry basket.
4. Cook the frittata for 8 minutes or until set. Serve and enjoy.

Nutrition:

- Calories: 384
- Fats: 23.3 g
- Carbs: 10.7 g
- Protein: 34.3 g

Omelet Frittata

Preparation Time: 10 minutes

Cooking Time: 6 minutes

Servings: 2

Ingredients:

- 3 eggs, lightly beaten

- 2 tbsp. cheddar cheese, shredded
- 2 tbsp. heavy cream
- 2 mushrooms, sliced
- ¼ small onion, chopped
- ¼ bell pepper, diced
- Pepper
- Salt

Directions:

1. In a bowl, whisk the eggs with the cream, vegetables, pepper, and salt.
2. Preheat the Air Fry Oven to 400ºF.
3. Pour the egg mixture into the sheet pan. Place the pan in the Air Fry Oven and cook for 5 minutes.
4. Add the shredded cheese on top of the frittata and cook for 1 minute more.
5. Serve and enjoy.

Nutrition:

- Calories: 160
- Fats: 10 g
- Carbs: 4 g
- Protein: 12 g

Cheese Soufflés

Preparation Time: 10 minutes
Cooking Time: 6 minutes
Servings: 8
Ingredients:

- 6 large eggs, separated
- ¾ cup heavy cream
- ¼ tsp. cayenne pepper
- ½ tsp. xanthan gum
- ½ tsp. pepper
- ¼ tsp. cream of tartar
- 2 tbsp. chives, chopped
- 2 cups cheddar cheese, shredded
- 1 tsp. salt
- 3 cups Almond flour

Directions:

1. Preheat the Air Fry Oven to 325ºF.
2. Spray 8 ramekins with cooking spray and set them aside.
3. In a bowl, whisk together the almond flour, cayenne pepper, pepper, salt, and xanthan gum.
4. Slowly add the heavy cream and mix to combine.

5. Whisk in the egg yolks, chives, and cheese until well combined.
6. In a large bowl, add the egg whites and tartar cream and beat until stiff peaks form.
7. Fold the egg white mixture into the almond flour mixture until combined.
8. Pour the mixture into the prepared ramekins. Divide the ramekins into batches.
9. Place the first batch of ramekins into the air fry basket.
10. Cook the soufflé for 20 minutes.
11. Serve and enjoy.

Nutrition:

- Calories: 210
- Fats: 16 g
- Carbs: 1 g
- Protein: 12 g

Simple Egg Soufflé

Preparation Time: 5 minutes
Cooking Time: 8 minutes
Servings: 2
Ingredients:

- 2 eggs
- ¼ tsp. chili pepper
- 2 tbsp. heavy cream
- ¼ tsp. pepper
- 1 tbsp. parsley, chopped
- Salt

Directions:

1. In a bowl, whisk the eggs with the remaining gradients.
2. Spray two ramekins with cooking spray.
3. Pour egg mixture into the prepared ramekins and place into the air fryer basket.
4. Cook the soufflé at 390ºF for 8 minutes.
5. Serve and enjoy.

Nutrition:

- Calories: 116
- Fats: 10 g
- Carbs: 1.1 g
- Protein: 6 g

Vegetable Egg Soufflé

Preparation Time: 10 minutes
Cooking Time: 20 minutes
Servings: 4

Ingredients:

- 4 large eggs
- 1 tsp. onion powder
- 1 tsp. garlic powder
- 1 tsp. red pepper, crushed
- ½ cup broccoli florets, chopped
- ½ cup mushrooms, chopped

Directions:

1. Sprinkle four ramekins with cooking spray and set them aside.
2. In a bowl, whisk the eggs with onion powder, garlic powder, and red pepper.
3. Add the mushrooms and broccoli and stir well.
4. Pour the egg mixture into the prepared ramekins and place the ramekins into the air fry basket.
5. Cook at 350ºF for 15 minutes. Make sure the soufflé is cooked; if the soufflé is not cooked, then cook for 5 minutes more.
6. Serve and enjoy.

Nutrition:

- Calories: 91
- Fats: 5.1 g
- Carbs: 4.7 g
- Protein 7.4 g

Asparagus Frittata

Preparation Time: 10 minutes
Cooking Time: 10 minutes
Servings: 4
Ingredients:

- 6 eggs
- 3 mushrooms, sliced
- 10 asparagus, chopped
- ¼ cup half and half
- 2 tsp. butter, melted
- 1 tsp. pepper
- 1 tsp. salt

Directions:

1. Toss the mushrooms and asparagus with the melted butter and add them into the air fry basket. Cook mushrooms and asparagus at 350ºF for 5 minutes Shake basket twice.
2. Meanwhile, in a bowl, whisk together eggs, half and half, pepper, and salt. Transfer the cooked mushrooms and asparagus into the sheet pan. Pour the egg mixture over mushrooms and asparagus.
3. Place the sheet pan in the Air Fry Oven and cook at 350ºF for 5 minutes, or until eggs are set. Slice and serve.

Nutrition:

- Calories: 211
- Fats: 13 g
- Carbs: 4 g
- Protein: 16 g

Spicy Cauliflower Rice

Preparation Time: 10 minutes
Cooking Time: 22 minutes
Servings: 2
Ingredients:

- 1 cauliflower head, cut into florets
- ½ tsp. cumin
- ½ tsp. chili powder
- 6 onion spring, chopped
- 2 jalapeños, chopped
- 4 tbsp. olive oil
- 1 zucchini, trimmed and cut into cubes
- ½ tsp. paprika
- ½ tsp. garlic powder
- ½ tsp. cayenne pepper
- ½ tsp. pepper
- ½ tsp. salt

Directions:

1. Preheat the air fryer to 370ºF.
2. Add the cauliflower florets into the food processor and process until it looks like rice.
3. Transfer the cauliflower rice onto the sheet pan and drizzle with half of the oil.
4. Place the sheet pan in the Air Fry Oven and cook for 12 minutes, stir halfway through.
5. Heat the remaining oil in a small pan over medium heat.
6. Add the zucchini and cook for 5–8 minutes
7. Add the onion and jalapeños and cook for 5 minutes.
8. Add the spices and stir well. Set aside.
9. Add the cauliflower rice to the zucchini mixture and stir well.
10. Serve and enjoy.

Nutrition:

- Calories: 254

- Fats: 28 g
- Carbs: 12.3 g
- Protein: 4.3 g

Broccoli Stuffed Peppers

Preparation Time: 10 minutes
Cooking Time: 40 minutes
Servings: 2
Ingredients:

- 4 eggs
- ½ cup cheddar cheese, grated
- 2 bell peppers cut in half and remove seeds
- ½ tsp. garlic powder
- 1 tsp. dried thyme
- ¼ cup feta cheese, crumbled
- ½ cup broccoli, cooked
- ¼ tsp. pepper
- ½ tsp. salt

Directions:

1. Preheat the Air Fry Oven to 325ºF.
2. In a bowl, beat the eggs and mix them with the seasonings, then pour the egg mixture into the pepper halves over feta and broccoli.
3. Place the bell pepper halves into the air fry basket and cook for 35–40 minutes.
4. Top with the grated cheddar cheese and cook until the cheese is melted.
5. Serve and enjoy.

Nutrition:

- Calories: 340
- Fats: 22 g
- Carbs: 12 g
- Protein: 22 g

Zucchini Muffins

Preparation Time: 10 minutes
Cooking Time: 20 minutes
Servings: 8
Ingredients:

- 6 eggs
- 4 drops stevia
- ¼ cup Swerve®
- ⅓ cup coconut oil, melted
- 1 cup zucchini, grated
- ¾ cup coconut flour
- ¼ tsp. ground nutmeg
- 1 tsp. ground cinnamon

- ½ tsp. baking soda

Directions:

1. Preheat the air fryer to 325ºF.
2. Add all the ingredients except the zucchini in a bowl and mix well.
3. Add the zucchini and stir well.
4. Pour the batter into the silicone muffin molds and place into the air fry basket.
5. Cook the muffins for 20 minutes.
6. Serve and enjoy.

Nutrition:

- Calories: 136
- Fats: 12 g
- Carbs: 1 g
- Protein: 4 g

Jalapeño Breakfast Muffins

Preparation Time: 10 minutes
Cooking Time: 15 minutes
Servings: 8
Ingredients:

- 5 eggs
- ⅓ cup coconut oil, melted
- 2 tsp. baking powder
- 3 tbsp. erythritol
- 3 tbsp. jalapeños, sliced
- ¼ cup unsweetened coconut milk
- 2/3 cup coconut flour
- ¾ tsp. sea salt

Directions:

1. Preheat the air fryer to 325ºF.
2. In a large bowl, mix together the coconut flour, baking powder, erythritol, and sea salt.
3. Stir in the eggs, jalapeños, coconut milk, and coconut oil until well combined.
4. Pour the batter into the silicone muffin molds and place into the air fry basket.
5. Cook muffins for 15 minutes.
6. Serve and enjoy.

Nutrition:

- Calories: 125
- Fats: 12 g
- Carbs: 7 g
- Protein: 3 g

Zucchini Noodles

Preparation Time: 10 minutes

Cooking Time: 44 minutes
Servings: 3
Ingredients:

- 1 egg
- ½ cup parmesan cheese, grated
- ½ cup feta cheese, crumbled
- 1 tbsp. thyme
- 1 garlic clove, chopped
- 1 onion, chopped
- 2 medium zucchinis, trimmed and spiralized
- 2 tbsp. olive oil
- 1 cup mozzarella cheese, grated
- ½ tsp. pepper
- ½ tsp. salt

Directions:

1. Preheat the air fryer to 350ºF.
2. Add the spiralized zucchini and salt to a colander and set aside for 10 minutes. Wash the zucchini noodles and pat dry with a paper towel.
3. Heat the oil in a pan over medium heat. Add the garlic and onion and sauté for 3–4 minutes.
4. Add the zucchini noodles and cook for 4–5 minutes or until softened.
5. Add the zucchini mixture into the air fryer baking pan. Add the egg, thyme, cheeses. Mix well and season.
6. Place the pan in the air fryer and cook for 30–35 minutes.
7. Serve and enjoy.

Nutrition:

- Calories: 435
- Fats: 29 g
- Carbs: 10.4 g
- Protein: 25 g

Mushroom Frittata

Preparation Time: 10 minutes
Cooking Time: 13 minutes
Servings: 1
Ingredients:

- 1 cup egg whites
- 1 cup spinach, chopped
- 2 mushrooms, sliced
- 2 tbsp. parmesan cheese, grated
- Salt

Directions:

1. Sprinkle the sheet pan with cooking spray and place it in the Air Fry Oven on medium heat. Add the mushrooms and sauté for 2–3 minutes. Add the spinach and cook for 1–2 minutes, or until wilted.
2. Transfer the mushroom spinach mixture to the sheet pan. Beat the egg whites in a mixing bowl until frothy. Season it with a pinch of salt.
3. Pour the egg white mixture into the spinach and mushroom mixture and sprinkle with parmesan cheese. Place the pan in Air Fry Oven and cook the frittata at 350ºF for 8 minutes.
4. Slice and serve.

Nutrition:

- Calories: 176
- Fats: 3 g
- Carbs: 4 g
- Protein: 31 g

Egg Muffins

Preparation Time: 10 minutes
Cooking Time: 15 minutes
Servings: 12
Ingredients:

- 9 eggs
- ½ cup onion, sliced
- 1 tbsp. olive oil
- 8 oz. ground sausage
- ¼ cup coconut milk
- ½ tsp. oregano
- 1 ½ cups spinach
- ¾ cup bell peppers, chopped
- Pepper
- Salt

Directions:

1. Preheat the Air Fry Oven to 325ºF.
2. Add the ground sausage in a pan and sauté over medium heat for 5 minutes.
3. Add the olive oil, oregano, bell pepper, and onion and sauté until the onion is translucent.
4. Put the spinach in the pan and cook for 30 seconds.
5. Remove pan from heat and set aside.
6. In a mixing bowl, whisk together the eggs, coconut milk, pepper, and salt until well beaten.
7. Add the sausage and vegetable mixture into the egg mixture and mix well.

8. Pour the egg mixture into the silicone muffin molds and place it into the air fry basket. (Cook in batches.)

9. Cook muffins for 15 minutes.

10. Serve and enjoy.

Nutrition:
- Calories: 135
- Fats: 11 g
- Carbs: 1.5 g
- Protein: 8 g

Blueberry Breakfast Cobbler

Preparation Time: 5 minutes
Cooking Time: 15 minutes
Servings: 4
Ingredients:
- ⅓ cup whole wheat pastry flour
- ¾ tsp. baking powder
- Dash sea salt
- ½ cup 2% milk
- 2 tbsp. pure maple syrup
- ½ tsp. vanilla extract
- Cooking oil spray
- ½ cup fresh blueberries
- ¼ cup granola, or plain store-bought granola

Directions:

1. In a medium bowl, whisk the flour, baking powder, and salt. Add the milk, maple syrup, and vanilla extract and gently whisk, just until thoroughly combined.

2. Preheat the Air Fry Oven by selecting "Bake" setting, the temperature to 350°F, and "Time" setting to 3 minutes. Select "Start/Pause" to start.

3. Spray a 6x6-inch round baking pan with cooking oil and pour the batter into the pan. Top evenly with the blueberries and granola.

4. Once the unit is preheated, place the pan into the air fry basket.

5. Select "Bake," set the temperature to 350°F, and set the time to 15 minutes. Select "Start/Pause" to begin.

6. When the cooking is complete, the cobbler should be nicely browned, and a knife inserted into the middle should come out clean. Enjoy plain or topped with a little vanilla yogurt.

Nutrition:

- Calories: 112
- Fats: 1 g
- Carbs: 23 g
- Protein: 3 g

Granola

Preparation Time: 5 minutes
Cooking Time: 40 minutes
Servings: 2
Ingredients:
- 1 cup rolled oats
- 3 tbsp. pure maple syrup
- 1 tbsp. sugar
- 1 tbsp. neutral-flavored oil, such as refined coconut, sunflower, or safflower
- ¼ tsp. sea salt
- ¼ tsp. ground cinnamon
- ¼ tsp. vanilla extract

Directions:

1. Insert the crisper plate into the air fry basket and the basket into the Air Fry Oven. Preheat it by selecting "Bake," setting the temperature to 250°F, and setting the time to 3 minutes. Select "Start/Pause" to start.

2. In a medium bowl, stir together the oats, maple syrup, sugar, oil, salt, cinnamon, and vanilla until thoroughly combined. Transfer the granola to a 6x6-inch round baking pan.

3. Once the unit is preheated, place the pan into the basket.

4. Select "Bake," set the temperature to 250°F and set the time to 40 minutes. Select "Start/Pause" to begin. After 10 minutes, stir the granola well. Resume cooking, stirring the granola every 10 minutes, for a total of 40 minutes, or until the granola is lightly browned and mostly dry.

5. Place the granola on a plate to cool. When the cooking is complete, it will become crisp as it cools. Store the completely cooled granola in an airtight container in a cool, dry place for 1 to 2 weeks.

Tip: You can change this recipe to include some of your favorite granola ingredients, such as dried fruits, different types of nuts, and even goodies such as chocolate chips. Stir them in after the granola is done, but before it's completely cool.

Nutrition:
- Calories: 165

- Fats: 5 g
- Carbs: 27 g
- Protein: 3 g

Mixed Berry Muffins

Preparation Time: 15 minutes
Cooking Time: 15 minutes
Servings: 8
Ingredients:

- 1 ⅓ cups plus 1 tbsp. all-purpose flour, divided
- ¼ cup granulated sugar
- 2 tbsp. light brown sugar
- 2 tsp. baking powder
- 2 eggs
- ⅔ cup whole milk
- ⅓ cup safflower oil
- 1 cup mixed fresh berries

Directions:

1. In a medium bowl, stir together 1 ⅓ cups of flour, the granulated sugar, brown sugar, and baking powder until mixed well.
2. In a small bowl, whisk the eggs, milk, and oil until combined. Mix the egg mixture into the dry ingredients just until combined.
3. In another small bowl, toss the mixed berries with the leftover flour until coated. Gently stir the berries into the batter.
4. Insert the crisper plate into the air fry basket and the basket into the Air Fry Oven. Preheat it by selecting "Bake," setting the temperature to 315°F, and setting the time to 3 minutes. Select "Start/Pause" to start.
5. Once the unit is preheated, place 4 cups into the basket and fill each ¾ full with the batter.
6. Select "Bake," set the temperature to 315°F, and set the time for 17 minutes. Select "Start/Pause" to begin.
7. After about 12 minutes, check the muffins. If they spring back when lightly touched with your finger, they are done. If not, resume cooking. When the cooking is done, transfer the muffins to a wire rack to cool. Repeat steps 6, 7, and 8 with the remaining muffin cups and batter. Let the muffins cool for 10 minutes before serving.

Nutrition:

- Calories: 230

Homemade Strawberry Breakfast Tarts

Preparation Time: 15 minutes
Cooking Time: 20 minutes
Servings: 6
Ingredients:

- 2 refrigerated piecrusts
- ½ cup strawberry preserves
- 1 tsp. cornstarch
- Cooking oil spray
- ½ cup low-Fat vanilla yogurt
- 1 oz. cream cheese, at room temperature
- 3 tbsp. confectioners' sugar
- Rainbow sprinkles for decorating

Directions:

1. Place the piecrusts on a flat surface. Cut each piecrust into 3 rectangles using a knife or pizza cutter, for 6 in total. Discard any unused dough from the piecrust edges.
2. In a small bowl, stir together the preserves and cornstarch. Mix well and ensure there are no lumps of cornstarch remaining.
3. Scoop 1 tbsp. of the strawberry mixture onto the top half of each piece of piecrust.
4. Fold the bottom of each piece up to enclose the filling. Press along the edges of each tart to seal using the back of a fork.
5. Insert the crisper plate into the basket and the air fry basket into the Air Fry Oven. Preheat it by selecting "Bake," setting the temperature to 375°F, and setting the time to 3 minutes Select "Start/Pause" to start.
6. Once the unit is preheated, spray the crisper plate with cooking oil. Work in batches, spray the breakfast tarts with cooking oil, and place them into the basket in a single layer. Do not stack the tarts.
7. Select "Bake," set the temperature to 375°F, and set the time to 10 minutes. Select "Start/Pause" to begin.
8. When the cooking is complete, the tarts should be light golden brown. Let the breakfast tarts cool fully before removing them from the air fry basket.

9. Repeat steps 5, 6, 7, and 8 for the remaining breakfast tarts.

10. In a small bowl, stir together the yogurt, cream cheese, and confectioners' sugar. Spread the breakfast tarts with the frosting and top with sprinkles.

Nutrition:
- Calories: 408
- Fats: 20.5 g
- Carbs: 56 g
- Protein: 1 g

Everything Bagels

Preparation Time: 10 minutes
Cooking Time: 10 minutes
Servings: 2
Ingredients:
- ½ cup self-rising flour, plus more for dusting
- ½ cup plain Greek yogurt
- 1 egg
- 1 tbsp. water
- 4 tsp. everything bagel spice mix
- Cooking oil spray
- 1 tbsp. butter, melted

Directions:
1. In a large bowl, and using a wooden spoon, stir together the flour and yogurt until a tacky dough forms. Transfer the dough to a lightly floured work surface and roll the dough into a ball.

2. Cut the dough into 2 pieces and roll each piece into a log. Form each log into a bagel shape, pinching the ends together.

3. In a small bowl, whisk the egg and water. Brush the egg wash on the bagels.

4. Sprinkle 2 tsp. of the spice mix on each bagel and gently press it into the dough.

5. Insert the crisper plate into the basket and the basket into the Air Fry Oven. Preheat it by selecting "Bake," setting the temperature to 330°F, and setting the time to 3 minutes. Select "Start/Pause" to begin.

6. Once the Air Fry Oven is hot enough, spray the crisper plate with cooking spray. Drizzle the bagels with the butter and place them into the basket.

7. Select "Bake," set the temperature to 330°F, and set the time to 10 minutes. Select "Start/Pause" to begin.

8. When the cooking is complete, the bagels should be lightly golden on the outside. Serve warm.

Nutrition:
- Calories: 271
- Fats: 13 g
- Carbs: 28 g
- Protein: 10 g

Easy Maple-Glazed Doughnuts

Preparation Time: 10 minutes
Cooking Time: 14 minutes
Servings: 8
Ingredients:
- 1 (8-count) can Jumbo® Flaky Biscuits
- Cooking oil spray
- ½ cup light brown sugar
- ¼ cup butter
- 3 tbsp. milk
- 2 cups confectioners' sugar, plus more for dusting (optional)
- 2 tsp. pure maple syrup

Directions:
1. Insert the crisper plate into the air fry basket and the basket into the Air Fry Oven. Preheat it by selecting "Air Fry," setting the temperature to 350°F, and setting the time to 3 minutes. Select "Start/Pause" to begin.

2. Remove the biscuits from the tube and cut out the center of each biscuit with a small, round cookie cutter.

3. Once the Ai Fry Oven is hot enough, spray the crisper plate with cooking oil. Work in batches, place 4 doughnuts into the basket.

4. Select "Air Fry," set the temperature to 350°F, and set the time to 5 minutes. Select "Start/Pause" to begin.

5. When the cooking is complete, place the doughnuts on a plate. Repeat steps 3 and 4 with the remaining doughnuts.

6. In a small saucepan over medium heat, combine the brown sugar, butter, and milk. Heat until the butter is melted, and the sugar is dissolved, about 4 minutes.

7.   Remove the pan from the heat and whisk in the confectioners' sugar and maple syrup until smooth.

8.   Dip the slightly cooled doughnuts into the maple sauce. Place them on a wire rack and dust with confectioners' sugar (if using). Let rest just until the sauce is set. Enjoy the doughnuts warm.

Nutrition:
- Calories: 219
- Fats: 10 g
- Carbs: 30 g
- Protein: 2 g

Chocolate-Filled Doughnut Holes

Preparation Time: 10 minutes
Cooking Time: 30 minutes
Servings: 12
Ingredients:
- 1 (8-count) can refrigerated biscuits
- Cooking oil spray
- 48 semisweet chocolate chips
- 3 tbsp. melted unsalted butter
- ¼ cup confectioners' sugar

Directions:

1.   Separate the biscuits and cut each biscuit into thirds for 24 pieces.

2.   Flatten each biscuit piece slightly and put 2 chocolate chips in the center of each. Wrap the dough around the chocolate and seal the edges well.

3.   Insert the crisper plate into the air fry basket and the basket into the Air Fry Oven. Preheat the unit by selecting air fry, setting the temperature to 330°F, and setting the time to 3 minutes Select "Start/Pause" to begin.

4.   Once the Air Fry Oven is hot enough, spray the crisper plate with cooking oil. Brush each doughnut hole with a bit of the butter and place it into the basket. Select "Air Fry," set the temperature to 330°F, and set the time between 8–12 minutes. Select "Start/Pause" to begin.

5.   The doughnuts are done when they are golden brown. When the cooking is complete, place the doughnut holes on a plate and dust with the confectioners' sugar. Serve warm.

Nutrition:
- Calories: 393
- Fats: 17 g

- Carbs: 55 g
- Protein: 5 g

Delicious Original Hash Browns

Preparation Time: 15 minutes
Cooking Time: 20 minutes
Servings: 4
Ingredients:
- 4 russet potatoes, peeled
- 1 tsp. paprika
- Salt
- Black pepper, freshly ground
- Cooking oil spray

Directions:

1.   Shred the potatoes with a box grater. If your grater has different hole sizes, use the largest ones.

2.   Place the shredded potatoes in a large bowl of cold water. Let it sit for 5 minutes (cold water helps remove excess starch from the potatoes.) Stir them to help dissolve the starch.

3.   Insert the crisper plate into the air fry basket and the basket into the Air Fry Oven. Preheat it by selecting "Air Fry," setting the temperature to 360°F, and setting the time to 3 minutes. Select "Start/Pause" to begin.

4.   Dry out the potatoes and pat them with paper towels until the potatoes are completely dry. Season the potatoes with paprika, salt, and pepper.

5.   Once the Air Fry Oven is hot enough, spray the crisper plate with cooking oil. Spray also the potatoes with the cooking oil and place them into the basket.

6.   Select "Air Fry," set the temperature to 360°F, and set the time to 20 minutes Select "Start/Pause" to begin.

7.   After 5 minutes, remove the basket and shake the potatoes. Reinsert the basket to resume cooking. Continue shaking the basket every 5 minutes (a total of 4 times), or until the potatoes are done.

8.   When the cooking is complete, remove the hash browns from the basket and serve warm.

Nutrition:
- Calories: 150
- Carbs: 34 g
- Protein: 4 g

Waffles and Chicken

Preparation Time: 15 minutes
Cooking Time: 30 minutes
Servings: 4
Ingredients:

- 8 whole chicken wings
- 1 tsp. garlic powder
- Chicken seasoning, for preparing the chicken
- Freshly ground black pepper
- ½ cup all-purpose flour
- Cooking oil spray
- 8 frozen waffles
- Pure maple syrup, for serving (optional)

Directions:

1. In a medium bowl, combine the chicken and garlic powder and season with chicken seasoning and pepper. Toss to coat.
2. Transfer the chicken to a resealable plastic bag and add the flour. Seal the bag and shake it to coat the chicken thoroughly.
3. Insert the crisper plate into the air fry basket and the basket into the unit. Preheat the unit by selecting "Air Fry," setting the temperature to 400°F, and setting the time to 3 minutes Select "Start/Pause" to begin.
4. Once the Air Fry Oven is hot enough, spray the crisper plate with cooking oil. Using tongs, transfer the chicken from the bag to the basket. (It is okay to stack the chicken wings on top of each other). Spray them with cooking oil.
5. Select "Air Fry," set the temperature to 400°F, and set the time to 20 minutes. Select "Start/Pause" to begin.
6. After 5 minutes, remove the basket and shake the wings. Reinsert the basket to resume cooking. Remove and shake the basket every 5 minutes until the chicken is fully cooked.
7. When the cooking is complete, remove the cooked chicken from the basket, and cover it to keep it warm.
8. Rinse the basket and crisper plate with warm water and insert it back into the Air Fry Oven.
9. Select "Air Fry," set the temperature to 360°F, and set the time to 3 minutes. Select "Start/Pause" to begin.
10. Once the Air Fry Oven is hot enough, spray the crisper plate with cooking spray. Work in batches, place the frozen waffles into the basket. Do not stack them. Spray the waffles with cooking oil.
11. Select "Air Fry," set the temperature to 360°F, and set the time to 6 minutes. Select "Start/Pause" to begin.
12. Repeat steps 10 and 11 with the remaining waffles when the cooking is complete.
13. Serve the waffles with the chicken, and a touch of maple syrup if desired.

Nutrition:

- Calories: 461
- Fats: 22 g
- Carbs: 45 g
- Protein: 28 g

Puffed Egg Tarts

Preparation Time: 10 minutes
Cooking Time: 20 minutes
Servings: 4
Ingredients:

- ⅓ sheet frozen puff pastry, thawed
- Cooking oil spray
- ½ cup shredded Cheddar cheese
- 2 eggs
- ¼ tsp. salt, divided
- 1 tsp. minced fresh parsley (optional)

Directions:

1. Insert the crisper plate into the air fry basket and the basket into the Air Fry Oven. Preheat it by selecting "Bake," setting the temperature to 390°F, and setting the time to 3 minutes. Select "Start/Pause" to begin.
2. Lay the puff pastry sheet on a piece of parchment paper and cut it in half.
3. Once the Air Fry Oven is hot enough, spray the crisper plate with cooking oil. Transfer the 2 squares of pastry to the basket, keeping them on the parchment paper.
4. Select "Bake," set the temperature to 390°F, and set the time to 20 minutes. Select "Start/Pause" to begin.
5. After 10 minutes, use a metal spoon to press down the center of each pastry square to make a sort of well. Divide the cheese equally between the baked pastries. Carefully, crack an egg on top of the

cheese, and sprinkle each with the salt. Resume cooking for 7–10 minutes.

6.   When the cooking is complete, the eggs will be cooked through. Sprinkle each with parsley (if using) and serve.

Nutrition:

- Calories: 322
- Fats: 24 g
- Carbs: 12 g
- Protein: 15 g

Early Morning Steak and Eggs

Preparation Time: 10 minutes
Cooking Time: 30 minutes
Servings: 4
Ingredients:

- Cooking oil spray
- 4 (4 oz.) New York strip steaks
- 1 tsp. granulated garlic, divided
- 1 tsp. salt, divided
- 1 tsp. freshly ground black pepper, divided
- 4 eggs
- ½ tsp. paprika

Directions:

1.   Insert the crisper plate into the air fry basket and the basket into the Air Fry Oven. Preheat it by selecting "Air Fry," setting the temperature to 360°F, and setting the time to 3 minutes. Select "Start/Pause" to begin.

2.   Once the unit is hot enough, spray the crisper plate with cooking oil. Place 2 steaks into the basket; do not oil or season them at this time.

3.   Select "Air Fry," set the temperature to 360°F, and set the time to 9 minutes. Select "Start/Pause" to begin.

4.   After 5 minutes, open the Air Fry Oven and flip the steaks. Sprinkle each with ¼ tsp. of granulated garlic, ¼ tsp. of salt, and ¼ tsp. of pepper. Resume cooking until the steaks register at least 145°F on a food thermometer.

5.   When the cooking is complete, transfer the steaks to a plate and tent with aluminum foil to keep warm. Repeat steps 2, 3, and 4 with the remaining steaks.

6.   Spray 4 ramekins with olive oil. Crack 1 egg into each ramekin. Sprinkle the eggs with the paprika

and the remaining ½ tsp. each of salt and pepper. Work in batches, place 2 ramekins into the basket.

7.   Select "Bake," set the temperature to 330°F, and set the time to 5 minutes. Select "Start/Pause" to begin. When the cooking is complete and the eggs are cooked to 160°F, remove the ramekins and repeat step 7 with the remaining 2 ramekins.

8.   Serve the eggs with the steaks.

Nutrition:

- Calories: 304
- Fats: 19 g
- Carbs: 2 g
- Protein: 31 g

Breakfast Potatoes

Preparation Time: 10 minutes
Cooking Time: 20 minutes
Serving: 6
Ingredients:

- 1 ½ tsp. olive oil, divided, plus more for misting
- 4 large potatoes, skin-on, cut into cubes
- 2 tsp. seasoned salt, divided
- 1 tsp. minced garlic, divided
- 2 large green or red bell peppers, cut into 1-inch pieces
- ½ onion, diced

Directions:

1.   Lightly, spray the air fryer basket with cooking oil.

2.   In a medium bowl, toss the potatoes with ½ tsp. of olive oil. Sprinkle with 1 tsp. of seasoned salt and ½ tsp. of minced garlic. Stir to coat.

3.   Place the seasoned potatoes in the fryer basket in a single layer.

4.   Cook for 5 minutes Shake the basket and cook for another 5 minutes

5.   Meanwhile, in a medium bowl, toss the bell peppers and onion with the remaining ½ tsp. of olive oil.

6.   Sprinkle the peppers and onions with the remaining 1 tsp. of seasoned salt and ½ tsp. of minced garlic. Stir to coat.

7.   Add the seasoned peppers and onions to the fryer basket with the potatoes.

8.   Cook for 5 minutes Shake the basket and cook for an additional 5 minutes

Nutrition:
- Calories: 199
- Fats: 1 g
- Carbs: 43 g
- Protein: 5 g

Baked Potato Breakfast Boats

Preparation Time: 10 minutes
Cooking Time: 20 minutes
Serving: 4
Ingredients:
- 2 large russet potatoes, scrubbed
- Olive oil
- Salt
- Black pepper, freshly ground
- 4 eggs
- 2 tbsp. chopped, cooked bacon
- 1 cup shredded cheddar cheese

Directions:
1. Poke holes in the potatoes with a fork and microwave on full power for 5 minutes. Turn potatoes over and cook for an additional 3–5 minutes, or until the potatoes are fork-tender.
2. Cut the potatoes in half lengthwise and use a spoon to scoop out the inside of the potato. Be careful to leave a layer of potato so that it makes a sturdy 'boat.' Lightly, spray the fry basket with olive oil. Spray the skin side of the potatoes with oil and sprinkle with salt and pepper to taste.
3. Place the potato skins in the fryer basket skin-side down. Crack one egg into each potato skin.
4. Sprinkle ½ tbsp. of bacon pieces and ¼ cup of shredded cheese on top of each egg. Sprinkle with salt and pepper to taste.
5. Air fry until the yolk is slightly runny, 5–6 minutes, or until the yolk is fully cooked, 7–10 minutes.

Nutrition:
- Calories: 338
- Fats: 15 g
- Saturated Fat: 8 g
- Cholesterol: 214 mg
- Carbs: 35 g
- Protein: 17 g
- Fiber: 3 g
- Sodium: 301 mg

Greek Frittata

Preparation Time: 10 minutes
Cooking Time: 20 minutes
Serving: 4
Ingredients:
- Olive oil
- 5 eggs
- ¼ tsp. salt
- ⅛ tsp. freshly ground black pepper
- 1 cup baby spinach leaves, shredded
- ½ cup halved grape tomatoes
- ½ cup crumbled feta cheese

Directions:
1. Spray a small round air fryer-friendly pan with olive oil.
2. In a medium bowl, whisk together the eggs, salt, and pepper and whisk to combine.
3. Add the spinach and stir to combine.
4. Pour ½ cup of the egg mixture into the pan.
5. Sprinkle ¼ cup of the tomatoes and ¼ cup of the feta on top of the egg mixture.
6. Cover the pan with aluminum foil and secure it around the edges.
7. Place the pan carefully into the fryer basket.
8. Air-fry for 12 minutes.
9. Remove the foil from the pan and cook until the eggs are set, 5–7 minutes.
10. Remove the frittata from the pan and place on a serving platter. Repeat with the remaining ingredients.

Nutrition:
- Calories: 146
- Fats: 10 g
- Saturated Fats: 5 g
- Cholesterol: 249 mg
- Carbs: 3 g
- Protein: 11 g
- Fiber: 1 g
- Sodium: 454 mg

Mini Shrimp Frittata

Preparation Time: 15 minutes
Cooking Time: 20 minutes
Serving: 4
Ingredients:
- 1 tsp. olive oil, plus more for spraying

- ½ small red bell pepper, finely diced
- 1 tsp. minced garlic
- 1 (4-oz.) can of tiny shrimp, dried out
- Salt
- Black pepper, freshly ground
- 4 eggs, beaten
- 4 tsp. ricotta cheese

Directions:

1.   Spray four ramekins with olive oil. Heat 1 tsp. of oil in a medium skillet over medium-high heat. Add the bell pepper and garlic and sauté until the pepper is soft, about 5 minutes.

2.   Add the shrimp, season with salt and pepper for 5–7 minutes, or until soft. Remove from the heat.

3.   Add the eggs and stir to combine. Pour one-quarter of the mixture into each ramekin.

4.   Place 2 ramekins in the fry basket and cook for 6 minutes. Remove the fryer basket from the Air Fry Oven and stir the mixture in each ramekin. Top each frittata with 1 tsp. of ricotta cheese. Return the basket to the Air Fry Oven and cook until eggs are set, and the top is lightly browned, about 4–5 minutes.

5.   Repeat with the remaining two ramekins.

Nutrition:

- Calories: 114
- Fats: 7 g
- Carbs: 1 g
- Protein: 12 g

Spinach and Mushroom Mini Quiche

Preparation Time: 10 minutes
Cooking Time: 15 minutes
Serving: 4
Ingredients:

- 1 tsp. olive oil, plus more for spraying
- 1 cup coarsely chopped mushrooms
- 1 cup fresh baby spinach, shredded
- 4 eggs, beaten
- ½ cup shredded Cheddar cheese
- ½ cup shredded mozzarella cheese
- ¼ tsp. salt
- ¼ tsp. black pepper

Directions:

1.   Spray 4 silicone baking cups with olive oil and set aside. In a medium sauté pan over medium

heat, warm 1 tsp. of olive oil. Add the mushrooms and sauté until soft, 3 to 4 minutes.

2.   Add the spinach and cook until wilted, 1–2 minutes Set aside.

3.   In a medium bowl, whisk together the eggs, Cheddar cheese, mozzarella cheese, salt, and pepper. Gently fold the mushrooms and spinach into the egg mixture.

4.   Pour ¼ of the mixture into each silicone baking cup. Place the baking cups into the fryer basket and air fry for 5 minutes Stir the mixture in each ramekin slightly and air fry until the egg has set, an additional 3–5 minutes.

Nutrition:

- Calories: 183
- Fats: 13 g
- Saturated Fats: 7 g
- Cholesterol: 206 mg
- Carbs: 3 g
- Protein: 14 g
- Fiber: 1 g
- Sodium: 411 mg

Italian Egg Cups

Preparation Time: 5 minutes
Cooking Time: 10 minutes
Serving: 4
Ingredients:

- Olive oil
- 1 cup marinara sauce
- 4 eggs
- 4 tbsp. shredded mozzarella cheese
- 4 tsp. grated Parmesan cheese
- Salt
- Freshly ground black pepper
- Chopped fresh basil, for garnish

Directions:

1.   Lightly, spray 4 individual ramekins with olive oil.

2.   Pour ¼ cup of marinara sauce into each ramekin.

3.   Crack 1 egg into each ramekin on top of the marinara sauce.

4.   Sprinkle 1 tbsp. of mozzarella and 1 tbsp. of Parmesan on top of each egg. Season it with salt and pepper.

5. Cover each ramekin with aluminum foil. Place 2 of the ramekins in the air fry basket.

6. Air-fry for 5 minutes and remove the aluminum foil. Air-fry until the top is lightly browned and the egg white is cooked, another 2–4 minutes. If you prefer the yolk to be firmer, cook for 3 to 5 more minutes.

7. Repeat with the remaining 2 ramekins. Garnish with the basil and serve.

Nutrition:
- Calories: 135
- Fats: 8 g
- Saturated Fats: 3 g
- Cholesterol: 191 mg
- Carbs: 6 g
- Protein: 10 g
- Fiber: 1 g
- Sodium: 407 mg

Mexican Breakfast Pepper Rings

Preparation Time: 5 minutes
Cooking Time: 10 minutes
Serving: 4
Ingredients:
- Olive oil
- 1 large red, yellow, or orange bell pepper, cut into four ¾-inch rings
- 4 eggs
- Salt
- Black pepper, freshly ground
- 2 tsp. salsa

Directions:
1. Lightly, spray a small round air fryer–friendly pan with olive oil.

2. Place 2 bell pepper rings on the pan. Crack 1 egg into each bell pepper ring. Season with salt and black pepper.

3. Spoon ½ tsp. of salsa on top of each egg. Place the pan in the fryer basket. Air-fry until the yolks are slightly runny, about 5–6 minutes, or until the yolks are fully cooked, 8–10 minutes.

4. Repeat with the remaining 2 pepper rings. Serve hot.

5. Pair it with turkey sausage or turkey bacon to make this a healthier morning meal.

Tip: To air-fry like a pro, use a silicone spatula to easily move the rings from the pan to your plate.

Nutrition:
- Calories: 84
- Fats: 5 g
- Saturated Fats: 2 g
- Cholesterol: 186 mg
- Carbs: 3 g
- Protein: 7 g
- Fiber: 1 g
- Sodium: 83 mg

Cajun Breakfast Muffins

Preparation Time: 10 minutes
Cooking Time: 10 minutes
Serving: 6
Ingredients:
- Olive oil
- 4 eggs, beaten
- 2 ¼ cups frozen hash browns, thawed
- 1 cup diced ham
- ½ cup shredded Cheddar cheese
- ½ tsp. Cajun seasoning

Directions:
1. Lightly spray 12 silicone muffin cups with olive oil.

2. In a medium bowl, mix together the eggs, hash browns, ham, Cheddar cheese, and Cajun seasoning.

3. Spoon 1 ½ tbsp. of the hash brown mixture into each muffin cup.

4. Place the muffin cups in the air fry basket.

5. Air-fry until the muffins are golden brown on top and the center has set up, about 8–10 minutes.

Tip: To make it even lower in calories, reduce or eliminate the cheese.

Nutrition:
- Calories: 178
- Fats: 9 g
- Saturated Fats: 4 g
- Cholesterol: 145 mg
- Carbs: 13 g
- Protein: 11 g
- Fiber: 2 g
- Sodium: 467 mg

Hearty Blueberry Oatmeal

Preparation Time: 10 minutes
Cooking Time: 25 minutes

Serving: 6

Ingredients:

- 1 ½ cups quick oats
- 1¼ tsp. ground cinnamon, divided
- ½ tsp. baking powder
- A Pinch salt
- 1 cup unsweetened vanilla almond milk
- ¼ cup honey
- 1 tsp. vanilla extract
- 1 egg, beaten
- 2 cups blueberries
- Olive oil
- 1 ½ tsp. sugar, divided
- 6 tbsp. low-Fat whipped topping (optional)

Directions:

1. In a large bowl, mix together the oats, 1 tsp. of cinnamon, baking powder, and salt.
2. In a medium bowl, whisk together the almond milk, honey, vanilla and egg.
3. Pour the liquid ingredients into the oats mixture and stir to combine. Fold in the blueberries.
4. Lightly, spray a round air fryer–friendly pan with oil.
5. Add half the blueberry mixture to the pan.
6. Sprinkle ⅛ tsp. of cinnamon and ½ tsp. of sugar over the top.
7. Cover the pan with aluminum foil and place gently in the air fry basket. Air-fry for 20 minutes remove the foil and air fry for an additional 5 minutes Transfer the mixture to a shallow bowl.
8. Repeat with the remaining blueberry mixture, ½ tsp. of sugar, and ⅛ tsp. of cinnamon.
9. To serve, spoon into bowls and top with the whipped topping.

Nutrition:

- Calories: 170
- Fats: 3 g
- Saturated Fats: 1 g
- Cholesterol: 97 mg
- Carbs: 34 g
- Protein: 4 g
- Fiber: 4 g
- Sodium: 97 mg

CHAPTER 3: LUNCH

Juicy Pork Chops

Preparation Time: 10 minutes
Cooking Time: 16 minutes
Servings: 4
Ingredients:

- 4 pork chops, boneless
- 2 tsp. olive oil
- ½ tsp. celery seed
- ½ tsp. parsley
- ½ tsp. granulated onion
- ½ tsp. granulated garlic
- ¼ tsp. sugar
- ½ tsp. salt

Directions:

1. In a small bowl, mix together the olive oil, celery seed, parsley, granulated onion, granulated garlic, sugar, and salt.
2. Rub the seasoning mixture all over the pork chops.
3. Place the pork chops on the sheet pan and cook at 350°F for 8 minutes.
4. Turn the pork chops to the other side and cook for 8 minutes more.
5. Serve and enjoy.

Nutrition:

- Calories: 279
- Fats: 22.3 g
- Carbs: 0.6 g
- Protein: 18.1 g

Crispy Meatballs

Preparation Time: 10 minutes
Cooking Time: 12 minutes
Servings: 8
Ingredients:

- 1 lb. ground pork
- 1 lb. ground beef
- 1 tbsp. Worcestershire sauce
- ½ cup feta cheese, crumbled
- ½ cup breadcrumbs
- 2 eggs, lightly beaten
- ¼ cup fresh parsley, chopped
- 1 tbsp. garlic, minced
- 1 onion, chopped

- ¼ tsp. pepper
- 1 tsp. salt

Directions:

1. Add all the ingredients into the mixing bowl and mix until well combined.
2. Spray the sheet pan with cooking spray.
3. Make small balls from the meat mixture and arrange them on a pan and air-fry at 400°F for 10–12 minutes.
4. Serve and enjoy.

Nutrition:

- Calories: 263
- Fats: 9 g
- Carbs: 7.5 g
- Protein: 35.9 g

Flavorful Steak

Preparation Time: 10 minutes
Cooking Time: 18 minutes
Servings: 2
Ingredients:

- 2 steaks, rinsed and pat dry
- ½ tsp. garlic powder
- 1 tsp. olive oil
- Pepper
- Salt

Directions:

1. Rub the steaks with olive oil and season with garlic powder, pepper, and salt.
2. Preheat the ninja foodi digital air fryer oven to 400°F.
3. Place the steaks on the air fryer oven pan and air-fry for 10–18 minutes, turning halfway through.
4. Serve and enjoy.

Nutrition:

- Calories: 361
- Fats: 10.9 g
- Carbs: 0.5 g
- Protein: 61.6 g

Lemon Garlic Lamb Chops

Preparation Time: 10 minutes
Cooking Time: 6 minutes
Servings: 6

Ingredients:

- 6 lamb loin chops
- 2 tbsp. fresh lemon juice
- 1 ½ tbsp. lemon zest
- 1 tbsp. dried rosemary
- 1 tbsp. olive oil
- 1 tbsp. garlic, minced
- Pepper
- Salt

Directions:

1.   Add the lamb chops to a mixing bowl. Add the remaining ingredients on top of the lamb chops and coat well.
2.   Arrange the lamb chops on Air Fry Oven tray and air fry at 400°F for 3 minutes. Turn lamb chops to another side and air-fry for 3 minutes more.
3.   Serve and enjoy.

Nutrition:

- Calories: 69
- Fats: 6 g
- Carbs: 1.2 g
- Protein: 3 g

Honey Mustard Pork Tenderloin

Preparation Time: 10 minutes
Cooking Time: 26 minutes
Servings: 4
Ingredients:

- 1 lb. pork tenderloin
- 1 tsp. sriracha sauce
- 1 tbsp. garlic, minced
- 2 tbsp. soy sauce
- 1 ½ tbsp. honey
- ¾ tbsp. Dijon mustard
- 1 tbsp. mustard

Directions:

1.   Add the sriracha sauce, garlic, soy sauce, honey, Dijon mustard, and mustard into a large Ziploc® bag and mix well.
2.   Add the pork tenderloin into the bag. Seal bag and place it in the refrigerator overnight. Preheat the ninja foodi digital air fryer oven to 380°F. Spray the ninja foodi digital air fryer tray with cooking spray, then place the marinated pork tenderloin on a tray and air-fry for 26 minutes. Turn the pork tenderloin after every 5 minutes. Slice and serve.

Nutrition:

- Calories: 195
- Fats: 4.1 g
- Carbs: 8 g
- Protein: 30.5 g

Easy Rosemary Lamb Chops

Preparation Time: 10 minutes
Cooking Time: 6 minutes
Servings: 4
Ingredients:

- 4 lamb chops
- 2 tbsp. dried rosemary
- ¼ cup fresh lemon juice
- Pepper
- Salt

Directions:

1.   In a small bowl, mix together the lemon juice, rosemary, pepper, and salt. Brush the lemon juice rosemary mixture over the lamb chops.
2.   Place the lamb chops in the air fry basket and air-fry at 400°F for 3 minutes. Turn the lamb chops to the other side and cook for 3 minutes more. Serve and enjoy.

Nutrition:

- Calories: 267
- Fats: 21.7 g
- Carbs: 1.4 g
- Protein: 16.9 g

BBQ Pork Ribs

Preparation Time: 10 minutes
Cooking Time: 12 minutes
Servings: 6
Ingredients:

- 1 slab baby back pork ribs, cut into pieces
- ½ cup BBQ sauce
- ½ tsp. paprika
- Salt

Directions:

1.   Add the pork ribs in a mixing bowl. Add the BBQ sauce, paprika, and salt over the pork ribs, coat them well and set aside for 30 minutes.
2.   Preheat the ninja foodi digital air fryer oven to 350°F. Arrange the marinated pork ribs in the ninja foodi digital air fryer oven pan and cook for 10–12 minutes, turning halfway through.
3.   Serve and enjoy.

Nutrition:
- Calories: 145
- Fats: 7 g
- Carbs: 10 g
- Protein: 9 g

Juicy Steak Bites

Preparation Time: 10 minutes
Cooking Time: 9 minutes
Servings: 4
Ingredients:
- 1 lb. sirloin steak, cut into bite-size pieces
- 1 tbsp. steak seasoning
- 1 tbsp. olive oil
- Pepper
- Salt

Directions:
1. Preheat the ninja foodi digital air fryer oven to 390°F.
2. Add the steak pieces into a large mixing bowl. Add the steak seasoning, oil, pepper, and salt over steak pieces and toss until well coated.
3. Transfer the steak pieces in the ninja foodi digital air fryer pan and air-fry for 5 minutes.
4. Turn the steak pieces to the other side and cook for 4 minutes more.
5. Serve and enjoy.

Nutrition:
- Calories: 241
- Fats: 10.6 g
- Protein: 34.4 g

Greek Lamb Chops

Preparation Time: 10 minutes
Cooking Time: 10 minutes
Servings: 4
Ingredients:
- 2 lbs. lamb chops
- 2 tsp. garlic, minced
- 1 ½ tsp. dried oregano
- ¼ cup fresh lemon juice
- ¼ cup olive oil
- ½ tsp. pepper
- 1 tsp. salt

Directions:

1. Add the lamb chops in a mixing bowl. Add the remaining ingredients over the lamb chops and coat well.
2. Arrange the lamb chops on the air fry basket and cook at 400°F for 5 minutes.
3. Turn the lamb chops and cook for 5 minutes more.
4. Serve and enjoy.

Nutrition:
- Calories: 538
- Fats: 29.4 g
- Carbs: 1.3 g
- Protein: 64 g

Easy Beef Roast

Preparation Time: 10 minutes
Cooking Time: 45 minutes
Servings: 6
Ingredients:
- 2 ½ lb. beef roast
- 2 tbsp. Italian seasoning

Directions:
1. Arrange the roast on the rotisserie spite.
2. Rub the roast with the Italian seasoning then insert into the the ninja foodi digital air fryer oven.
3. Air-fry at 350°F for 45 minutes or until the internal temperature of the roast reaches 145°F.
4. Slice and serve.

Nutrition:
- Calories: 365
- Fats: 13.2 g
- Carbs: 0.5 g
- Protein: 57.4 g

Herb Butter Rib Eye Steak

Preparation Time: 10 minutes
Cooking Time: 14 minutes
Servings: 4
Ingredients:
- 2 lb. rib eye steak, bone-in
- 1 tsp. fresh rosemary, chopped
- 1 tsp. fresh thyme, chopped
- 1 tsp. fresh chives, chopped
- 2 tsp. fresh parsley, chopped
- 1 tsp. garlic, minced
- ¼ cup butter softened

- Pepper
- Salt

Directions:

1. In a small bowl, combine together the butter and the herbs.
2. Rub the herb-butter mixture on the rib eye steak and place it in the refrigerator for 30 minutes.
3. Place the marinated steak in the ninja foodi digital air fryer oven pan and cook at 400°F for 12–14 minutes.
4. Serve and enjoy.

Nutrition:

- Calories: 416
- Fats: 36.7 g
- Carbs: 0.7 g
- Protein: 20.3 g

Classic Beef Jerky

Preparation Time: 10 minutes
Cooking Time: 4 hours
Servings: 4
Ingredients:

- 2 lbs. London broil, sliced thinly
- 1 tsp. onion powder
- 3 tbsp. brown sugar
- 3 tbsp. soy sauce
- 1 tsp. olive oil
- ¾ tsp. garlic powder

Directions:

1. Add all the ingredients except the meat in a large Ziploc® bag.
2. Mix until well combined. Add the meat in the bag.
3. Seal the bag and massage gently to cover the meat with marinade.
4. Let the meat marinate for 1 hour.
5. Arrange the marinated meat slices in the ninja foodi digital air fryer tray and dehydrate at 160°F for 4 hours.

Nutrition:

- Calories: 133
- Fats: 4.7 g
- Carbs: 9.4 g
- Protein: 13.4 g

BBQ Pork Chops

Preparation Time: 10 minutes

Cooking Time: 7 minutes
Servings: 4
Ingredients:

- 4 pork chops

For the Rub:

- ½ tsp. allspice
- ½ tsp. dry mustard
- 1 tsp. ground cumin
- 1 tsp. garlic powder
- ½ tsp. chili powder
- ½ tsp. paprika
- 1 tbsp. brown sugar
- 1 tsp salt

Directions:

1. In a small bowl, mix together all the rub ingredients and rub all over the pork chops.
2. Arrange the pork chops in the air fry basket and air-fry at 400°F for 5 minutes.
3. Turn the pork chops to other side and air-fry for 2 minutes more.
4. Serve and enjoy.

Nutrition:

- Calories: 273
- Fats: 20.2 g
- Carbs: 3.4 g
- Protein: 18.4 g

Simple Beef Patties

Preparation Time: 10 minutes
Cooking Time: 13 minutes
Servings: 4
Ingredients:

- 1 lb. ground beef
- ½ tsp. garlic powder
- ¼ tsp. onion powder
- Pepper
- Salt

Directions:

1. Preheat the ninja foodi digital air fryer oven to 400°F.
2. Add the ground meat, garlic powder, onion powder, pepper, and salt into the mixing bowl and mix until well combined.
3. Make even-shaped patties from the meat mixture and arrange them in the air fryer pan.
4. Place the pan in the ninja foodi digital air fryer oven.

5. Cook the patties for 10 minutes Turn patties after 5 minutes.
6. Serve and enjoy.

Nutrition:
- Calories: 212
- Fats: 7.1 g
- Carbs: 0.4 g
- Protein: 34.5 g

Simple Beef Sirloin Roast

Preparation Time: 10 minutes
Cooking Time: 50 minutes
Servings: 8
Ingredients:
- 2 ½ lb. sirloin roast
- Salt and ground black pepper, as required

Directions:
1. Rub the roast with salt and black pepper generously.
2. Insert the rotisserie rod through the roast.
3. Insert the rotisserie forks, one on each side of the rod to secure the rod to the chicken.
4. Arrange the drip pan in the bottom of the Ninja foodi digital Plus Air Fryer Oven cooking chamber.
5. Select "Roast" and then adjust the temperature to 350°F.
6. Set the timer for 50 minutes and press "Start."
7. When the display shows "Add Food," press the red lever down and load the left side of the rod into the Ninja foodi digital air fryer.
8. Now, slide the rod's left side into the groove along the metal bar so it doesn't move. Then, close the door and touch "Rotate." Press the red lever to release the rod when cooking time is complete.
9. Remove from the Ninja foodi digital air fryer and place the roast onto a platter for about 10 minutes before slicing. With a sharp knife, cut the roast into the desired slice sizes and serve.

Nutrition:
- Calories: 201
- Fats: 8.8 g
- Protein: 28.9 g

Seasoned Beef Roast

Preparation Time: 10 minutes

Cooking Time: 45 minutes
Servings: 10
Ingredients:
- 3 lb. beef top roast
- 1 tbsp. olive oil
- 2 tbsp. Montreal steak seasoning

Directions:
1. Coat the roast with oil and then rub with the seasoning generously.
2. With the help of kitchen twines, tie the roast to keep it compact. Arrange the roast onto the cooking tray.
3. Arrange the drip pan in the bottom of the Ninja foodi digital plus Air Fryer Oven cooking chamber.
4. Select "Air Fry" and then adjust the temperature to 360°F. Set the timer for 45 minutes and press "Start."
5. When the display shows "Add Food," insert the cooking tray in the center position.
6. When the display shows "Turn Food," do nothing.
7. When cooking time is complete, remove the tray from Ninja foodi digital air fryer and place the roast onto a platter for about 10 minutes before slicing. With a sharp knife, cut the roast into desired slice sizes and serve.

Nutrition:
- Calories: 269
- Fats: 9.9 g

Bacon Wrapped Filet Mignon

Preparation Time: 10 minutes
Cooking Time: 15 minutes
Servings: 2
Ingredients:
- 2 bacon slices
- 2 (4-oz.) filet mignon
- Salt and ground black pepper, as required
- Olive oil cooking spray

Directions:
1. Wrap 1 bacon slice around each filet mignon and secure with toothpicks.
2. Season the filets lightly with the salt and black pepper.
3. Arrange the filet mignon onto a coking rack and spray with cooking spray.

4. Place the drip pan in the bottom of the Ninja foodi digital plus Air Fryer Oven cooking chamber.

5. Select "Air Fry" and then adjust the temperature to 375°F.

6. Set the timer for 15 minutes and press "Start."

7. When the display shows "Add Food," insert the cooking rack in the center position.

8. Turn the filets when the display shows "Turn Food."

9. When cooking time is complete, remove the rack from the Ninja foodi digital air fryer and serve hot.

Nutrition:
- Calories: 360
- Fats: 19.6 g
- Carbs: 0.4 g
- Protein: 42.6 g

Beef Burger

Preparation Time: 15 minutes
Cooking Time: 18 minutes
Servings: 4
Ingredients:
For the Burgers:
- 1 lb. ground beef
- ½ cup panko breadcrumbs
- ¼ cup onion, chopped finely
- 3 tbsp. Dijon mustard
- 3 tsp. low-sodium soy sauce
- 2 tsp. fresh rosemary, chopped finely
- Salt, to taste

For the Sauce:
- 2 tbsp. Dijon mustard
- 1 tbsp. brown sugar
- 1 tsp. soy sauce
- 4 slices Gruyére cheese

Directions:
1. In a large bowl, add all the ingredients and mix until well combined.

2. Make 4 equal-sized patties from the mixture.

3. Arrange the patties onto a cooking tray.

4. Arrange the drip pan in the bottom of the Ninja foodi digital Plus Air Fryer Oven cooking chamber.

5. Select "Air Fry" and then adjust the temperature to 370°F.

6. Set the timer for 15 minutes and press "Start."

7. When the display shows "Add Food" insert the cooking rack in the center position.

8. Turn the burgers when the display shows "Turn Food."

9. To make the sauce, add the mustard, brown sugar and soy sauce and mix well.

10. When cooking time is complete, remove the tray from the Ninja foodi digital air fryer and coat the burgers with the sauce.

11. Top each burger with 1 cheese slice.

12. Return the tray to the cooking chamber and select "Broil."

13. Set the timer for 3 minutes and press "Start."

14. When cooking time is complete, remove the tray from the Ninja foodi digital air fryer and serve hot.

Nutrition:
- Calories: 402 Fats: 18 g
- Carbs: 6.3 g
- Protein: 44.4 g

Season and Salt-Cured Beef

Preparation Time: 15 minutes
Cooking Time: 3 hours
Servings: 4
Ingredients:
- 1 ½ lb. beef round, trimmed
- ½ cup Worcestershire sauce
- ½ cup low-sodium soy sauce
- 2 tsp. honey
- 1 tsp. liquid smoke
- 2 tsp. onion powder
- ½ tsp. red pepper flakes
- Ground black pepper, as required

Directions:
1. In a ziploc® bag, place the beef and freeze for 1–2 hours.

2. Place the meat onto a cutting board and cut against the grain into ⅛–¼-inch strips.

3. In a large bowl, add the remaining ingredients and mix until well combined.

4. Add the steak slices and coat with the mixture generously.

5. Refrigerate to marinate for about 4-6 hours.

6. Remove the beef slices from the bowl and with paper towels, pat dry them.

7. Divide the steak strips onto the cooking trays and arrange in an even layer.

8. Select "Dehydrate" and then adjust the temperature to 160°F.

9. Set the timer for 3 hours and press "Start."

10. When the display shows "Add Food," insert 1 tray in the top position and another in the center position.

11. After 1 ½ hours, switch the position of cooking trays.

12. Meanwhile, in a small pan, add the remaining ingredients over medium heat and cook for about 10 minutes, stirring occasionally.

13. When cooking the time is complete, remove the trays from the Ninja foodi digital air fryer.

Nutrition:
- Calories: 372
- Fats: 10.7 g
- Carbs: 12 g
- Protein: 53.8 g

Sweet & Spicy Meatballs

Preparation Time: 20 minutes
Cooking Time: 30 minutes
Servings: 8
Ingredients:
For the Meatballs:
- 2 lb. lean ground beef
- 2/3 cup quick-cooking oats
- ½ cup Ritz® crackers, crushed
- 1 (5-oz.) can evaporated milk
- 2 large eggs, lightly beaten
- 1 tsp. honey
- 1 tbsp. dried onion, minced
- 1 tsp. garlic powder
- 1 tsp. ground cumin
- Salt and ground black pepper, as required

For the Sauce:
- ⅓ cup orange marmalade
- ⅓ cup honey
- ⅓ cup brown sugar
- 2 tbsp. cornstarch
- 2 tbsp. soy sauce
- 1-2 tbsp. hot sauce
- 1 tbsp. Worcestershire sauce

Directions:
1. To make the meat balls, add all the ingredients and mix until well combined.

2. Make 1 ½-inch balls from the mixture.

3. Arrange half of the meatballs onto a cooking tray in a single layer.

4. Arrange the drip pan in the bottom of the Ninja foodi digital Plus Air Fryer Oven cooking chamber.

5. Select "Air Fry" and then adjust the temperature to 380°F.

6. Set the timer for 15 minutes and press "Start."

7. When the display shows "Add Food," insert the cooking tray in the center position.

8. Turn the meat balls when the display shows "Turn Food."

9. When cooking time is complete, remove the tray from the Ninja foodi digital air fryer.

10. Repeat with the remaining meatballs.

11. To make the sauce, add all the ingredients in a small pan over medium heat and stir continuously.

12. Serve the meatballs with the sauce.

Nutrition:
- Calories: 411
- Fats: 11.1 g
- Carbs: 38.8 g
- Protein: 38.9 g

Spiced Pork Shoulder

Preparation Time: 15 minutes
Cooking Time: 55 minutes
Servings: 6
Ingredients:
- 1 tsp. ground cumin
- 1 tsp. cayenne pepper
- 1 tsp. garlic powder
- Salt and ground black pepper, as required
- 2 lb. pork shoulder, skin-on

Directions:
1. In a small bowl, mix together the spices, salt and black pepper.

2. Arrange the pork shoulder skin-side down on a cutting board.
3. Season the inner side of the pork shoulder with salt and black pepper.
4. With kitchen twines, tie the pork shoulder into a long round cylinder shape.
5. Season the outer side of the pork shoulder with the spice mixture.
6. Insert the rotisserie rod through the pork shoulder.
7. Insert 1 rotisserie fork on each side of the rod to secure the pork shoulder.
8. Arrange the drip pan in the bottom of the Ninja foodi digital Plus Air Fryer Oven cooking chamber.
9. Select "Roast" and then adjust the temperature to 350°F.
10. Set the timer for 55 minutes and press the "Start."
11. When the display shows "Add Food," press the red lever down and load the left side of the rod into the Ninja foodi digital air fryer.
12. Now slide the rod's left side into the groove along the metal bar so it doesn't move.
13. Then close the door and touch "Rotate."
14. Press the red lever to release the rod when cooking time is complete.
15. Remove the pork from the Ninja foodi digital air fryer and place onto a platter for about 10 minutes before slicing.
16. With a sharp knife, cut the pork shoulder into the desired slice sizes and serve.

Nutrition:
- Calories: 445
- Fats: 32.5 g
- Carbs: 0.7 g
- Protein: 35.4 g

Seasoned Pork Tenderloin

Preparation Time: 10 minutes
Cooking Time: 45 minutes
Servings: 5
Ingredients:
- 1 ½ lb. pork tenderloin
- 2–3 tbsp. BBQ pork seasoning

Directions:

1. Rub the pork with seasoning generously. Insert the rotisserie rod through the pork tenderloin.
2. Insert the rotisserie forks, one on each side of the rod to secure the pork tenderloin.
3. Arrange the drip pan in the bottom of the Ninja foodi digital plus Air Fryer Oven cooking chamber.
4. Select "Roast" and then adjust the temperature to 360 degrees F.
5. Set the timer for 45 minutes and press "Start."
6. When the display shows "Add Food," press the red lever down and load the left side of the rod into the Ninja foodi digital air fryer.
7. Now, slide the rod's left side into the groove along the metal bar so it doesn't move.
8. Then, close the door and touch "Rotate."
9. Press the red lever to release the rod when cooking time is complete.
10. Remove the pork from the Ninja foodi digital air fryer and place onto a platter for about 10 minutes before slicing.
11. With a sharp knife, cut the roast into desired slice sizes and serve.

Nutrition:
- Calories: 195
- Fats: 4.8 g
- Protein: 35.6 g

Garlicky Pork Tenderloin

Preparation Time: 15 minutes
Cooking Time: 20 minutes
Servings: 5
Ingredients:
- 1 ½ lb. pork tenderloin
- Non-stick cooking spray
- 2 small heads roasted garlic
- Salt and ground black pepper, as required

Directions:

1. Lightly, spray all the sides of pork with cooking spray and season with salt and black pepper.
2. Now, rub the pork with roasted garlic. Arrange the roast onto the lightly greased cooking tray.
3. Arrange the drip pan in the bottom of the Ninja foodi digital plus Air Fryer Oven cooking chamber.

4. Select "Air Fry" and then adjust the temperature to 400°F. Set the timer for 20 minutes and press the "Start."

5. When the display shows "Add Food" insert the cooking tray in the center position.

6. Turn the pork when the display shows "Turn Food."

7. When cooking time is complete, remove the tray from the Ninja foodi digital air fryer and place the pork onto a platter for about 10 minutes before slicing. With a sharp knife, cut the pork into desired slice sizes and serve.

Nutrition:
- Calories: 202
- Fats: 4.8 g
- Carbs: 1.7 g
- Protein: 35.9 g

Glazed Pork Tenderloin

Preparation Time: 15 minutes
Cooking Time: 20 minutes
Servings: 3
Ingredients:
- 1-lb. pork tenderloin
- 2 tbsp. Sriracha
- 2 tbsp. honey
- Salt, as required

Directions:
1. Insert the rotisserie rod through the pork tenderloin.

2. Insert 1 rotisserie fork on each side of the rod to secure the pork tenderloin.

3. In a small bowl, add the Sriracha, honey and salt and mix well.

4. Brush the pork tenderloin evenly with honey mixture.

5. Arrange the drip pan in the bottom of the Ninja foodi digital plus Air Fryer Oven cooking chamber.

6. Select "Air Fry" and then adjust the temperature to 350°F.

7. Set the timer for 20 minutes and press the "Start."

8. When the display shows "Add Food," press the red lever down and load the left side of the rod into the Ninja foodi digital air fryer.

9. Now, slide the rod's left side into the groove along the metal bar so it doesn't move.

10. Then, close the door and touch "Rotate."

11. Press the red lever to release the rod when cooking time is complete.

12. Remove the pork from the Ninja foodi digital air fryer and place onto a platter for about 10 minutes before slicing.

13. With a sharp knife, cut the pork into desired slice sizes and serve.

Nutrition:
- Calories: 269
- Fats: 5.3 g
- Carbs: 13.5 g
- Protein: 39.7 g

Country Style Pork Tenderloin

Preparation Time: 15 minutes
Cooking Time: 25 minutes
Servings: 3
Ingredients:
- 1 lb. pork tenderloin
- 1 tbsp. garlic, minced
- 2 tbsp. soy sauce
- 2 tbsp. honey
- 1 tbsp. Dijon mustard
- 1 tbsp. grain mustard
- 1 tsp. Sriracha sauce

Directions:
1. In a large bowl, add all the ingredients except the pork and mix well.

2. Add the pork tenderloin and coat with the mixture generously.

3. Refrigerate to marinate for 2–3 hours.

4. Remove the pork tenderloin from the bowl, reserving the marinade.

5. Place the pork tenderloin on a lightly greased cooking tray.

6. Arrange the drip pan in the bottom of the Ninja foodi digital plus Air Fryer Oven cooking chamber.

7. Select "Air Fry" and then adjust the temperature to 380°F.

8. Set the timer for 25 minutes and press the "Start."

9. When the display shows "Add Food," insert the cooking tray in the center position.

10.   Turn the pork when the display shows "Turn Food" and coat it with the reserved marinade.

11.   When cooking time is complete, remove the tray from the Ninja foodi digital air fryer and place the pork tenderloin onto a platter for about 10 minutes before slicing.

12.   With a sharp knife, cut the pork tenderloin into the desired slice sizes and serve.

Nutrition:
- Calories: 277
- Fats: 5.7 g
- Carbs: 14.2 g
- Protein: 40.7 g

Seasoned Pork Chops

Preparation Time: 10 minutes
Cooking Time: 12 minutes
Servings: 4
Ingredients:
- 4 (6-oz.) pork chops, boneless
- 2 tbsp. pork rub
- 1 tbsp. olive oil

Directions:

1.   Coat both sides of the pork chops with the oil and the pork rub.

2.   Place the pork chops onto the lightly greased cooking tray.

3.   Arrange the drip pan in the bottom of the Ninja foodi digital plus Air Fryer Oven cooking chamber.

4.   Select "Air Fry" and then adjust the temperature to 400°F.

5.   Set the timer for 12 minutes and press "Start."

6.   When the display shows "Add Food," insert the cooking tray in the center position.

7.   Turn the pork chops when the display shows "Turn Food."

8.   When cooking time is complete, remove the tray from the Ninja foodi digital air fryer and serve hot.

Nutrition:
- Calories: 285
- Fats: 9.5 g
- Carbs: 1.5 g
- Protein: 44.5 g

Breaded Pork Chops

Preparation Time: 15 minutes
Cooking Time: 28 minutes
Servings: 2
Ingredients:
- 2 (5-oz.) boneless pork chops
- 1 cup buttermilk
- ½ cup flour
- 1 tsp. garlic powder
- Salt and ground black pepper, as required
- Olive oil cooking spray

Directions:

1.   In a bowl, place the chops and buttermilk and refrigerate, covered for about 12 hours.

2.   Remove the chops from the bowl and discard the buttermilk.

3.   In a shallow dish, mix together the flour, garlic powder, salt, and black pepper.

4.   Coat the chops generously with flour mixture.

5.   Place the pork chops onto the cooking tray and spray with the cooking spray.

6.   Arrange the drip pan in the bottom of the Ninja foodi digital plus Air Fryer Oven cooking chamber.

7.   Select "Air Fry" and then adjust the temperature to 380°F.

8.   Set the timer for 28 minutes and press the "Start."

9.   When the display shows "Add Food," insert the cooking tray in the center position.

10.   Turn the pork chops when the display shows "Turn Food."

11.   When cooking time is complete, remove the tray from the Ninja foodi digital air fryer and serve hot.

Nutrition:
- Calories: 370
- Fats: 6.4 g
- Carbs: 30.7 g
- Protein: 44.6 g

Crusted Rack of Lamb

Preparation Time: 15 minutes
Cooking Time: 19 minutes **Servings:** 4
Ingredients:
- 1 rack of lamb, fat removed

- Salt and ground black pepper, as required
- ⅓ cup pistachios, chopped finely
- 2 tbsp. panko breadcrumbs
- 2 tsp. fresh thyme, chopped finely
- 1 tsp. fresh rosemary, chopped finely
- 1 tbsp. butter, melted
- 1 tbsp. Dijon mustard

Directions:

1. Insert the rotisserie rod through the rack on the meaty side of the ribs, right next to the bone.
2. Insert 1 rotisserie fork on each side of the rod to secure the rack.
3. Season the rack with salt and black pepper evenly.
4. Arrange the drip pan in the bottom of the Ninja foodi digital plus Air Fryer Oven cooking chamber.
5. Select "Air Fry" and then adjust the temperature to 380°F.
6. Set the timer for 12 minutes and press the "Start."
7. When the display shows "Add Food," press the red lever down and load the left side of the rod into the Ninja foodi digital air fryer.
8. Now slide the rod's left side into the groove along the metal bar so it doesn't move.
9. Then, close the door and touch "Rotate."
10. Mix together the remaining ingredients in a small bowl, except the mustard.
11. Press the red lever to release the rod when cooking time is complete.
12. Remove the rack from the Ninja foodi digital air fryer and brush the meaty side with the mustard.
13. Then coat the pistachio mixture on all sides of the rack and press firmly.
14. Now place the rack of lamb onto the cooking tray, meat side up.
15. Select "Air Fry" and adjust the temperature to 380°F.
16. Set the timer for 7 minutes and press the "Start."
17. When the display shows "Add Food," insert the cooking tray in the center position.
18. When the display shows "Turn Food" do nothing.
19. When cooking time is complete, remove the tray from the Ninja foodi digital air fryer and place the rack onto a cutting board for at least 10 minutes
20. Cut the rack into individual chops and serve.

Nutrition:

- Calories: 824 Fats: 39.3 g
- Carbs: 10.3 g Protein: 72 g

Lamb Burgers

Preparation Time: 15 minutes
Cooking Time: 8 minutes
Servings: 6
Ingredients:

- 2 lb. ground lamb
- 1 tbsp. onion powder
- Salt and ground black pepper, as required

Directions:

1. In a bowl, add all the ingredients and mix well.
2. Make 6 equal-sized patties from the mixture.
3. Arrange the patties on a cooking tray.
4. Arrange the drip pan in the bottom of Ninja foodi digital plus Air Fryer Oven cooking chamber.
5. Select "Air Fry" and then adjust the temperature to 360 degrees F.
6. Set the timer for 8 minutes and press "Start."
7. When the display shows "Add Food," insert the cooking rack in the center position.
8. Turn the burgers when the display shows "Turn Food."
9. When cooking time is complete, remove the tray from Ninja foodi digital air fryer and serve hot.

Nutrition:

- Calories: 285
- Fats: 11.1 g
- Carbs: 0.9 g
- Protein: 42.6 g

Salmon

Preparation Time: 5 minutes
Cooking Time: 12 minutes
Servings: 2
Ingredients

- 2 salmon fillets, wild-caught, each about 1 ½-inch thick

- 1 tsp. ground black pepper
- 2 tsp. paprika
- 1 tsp. salt
- 2 tsp. olive oil

Directions:

1. Switch the Air Fry Oven on, insert the basket, grease it with olive oil, close it and set it at 390ºF. Meanwhile, rub each salmon fillet with oil and then season with black pepper, paprika, and salt.

2. Open the , add seasoned salmon in it, close the Air Fry Oven and cook for 7 minutes, or until nicely golden and cooked, flipping the fillets halfway through the frying. When the Air Fry Oven beeps, open its lid and transfer the salmon onto a serving plate and serve.

Nutrition:

- Calories: 288
- Carbs: 1.4 g
- Fats: 18.9 g
- Protein: 28.3 g

Parmesan Shrimp

Preparation Time: 10 minutes
Cooking Time: 10 minutes
Servings: 6
Ingredients

- 2 lb. jumbo shrimp, wild-caught, peeled, deveined
- 2 tbsp. minced garlic
- 1 tsp. onion powder
- 1 tsp. basil
- 1 tsp. ground black pepper
- ½ tsp. dried oregano
- 2 tbsp. olive oil
- 2/3 cup grated parmesan cheese, reduced fat
- 2 tbsp. lemon juice

Directions:

1. Switch the Air Fry Oven on, insert the basket, grease it with olive oil, close it and set it at 350ºF.

2. Meanwhile, place the cheese in a bowl, add the remaining ingredients except the shrimps and the lemon juice, and stir until combined.

3. Add the shrimps and then toss until well coated.

4. Open the Air Fry Oven, add the shrimps, spray oil over them, close the Air Fry Oven and cook for 10 minutes, or until nicely golden and crispy, shaking halfway through the frying. When air fryer beeps, open its lid, transfer chicken onto a serving plate, and drizzle with lemon juice and serve.

Nutrition:

- Calories: 307
- Carbs: 12 g
- Fats: 16.4 g
- Protein: 27.6 g

Shrimp with Lemon and Chile

Preparation Time: 5 minutes
Cooking Time: 12 minutes
Servings: 2
Ingredients:

- 1 lb. shrimp, wild-caught, peeled, deveined
- 1 lemon, sliced
- 1 small red chili pepper, sliced
- ½ tsp. ground black pepper
- ½ tsp. garlic powder
- 1 tsp. salt
- 1 tbsp. olive oil

Directions:

1. Switch the Air Fry Oven on, insert the basket, grease it with olive oil, close it and set it at 400ºF.

2. Meanwhile, place the shrimps in a bowl, add the garlic, salt, black pepper, oil, and lemon slices and toss until combined. Open the Air Fry Oven, add shrimps and lemon in it, close it, and cook for 5 minutes, shaking halfway through the frying. Then add the chili slices, shake the basket until mixed and continue cooking for 2 minutes or until shrimps are opaque and crispy. When the Air Fry Oven beeps, open its lid, transfer shrimps and lemon slices onto a serving plate and serve.

Nutrition:

- Calories: 112.5
- Carbs: 1 g
- Fats: 1 g
- Protein: 2 g

Tilapia

Preparation Time: 5 minutes
Cooking Time: 12 minutes
Servings: 2
Ingredients:

- 2 tilapia fillets, wild-caught, 1 ½ inch thick
- 1 tsp. OLD BAY® seasoning
- ¾ tsp. lemon pepper seasoning
- ½ tsp. salt

Directions:

1. Switch the Air Fry Oven on, insert the basket, grease it with olive oil, close it and set it at 400ºF.

2. Meanwhile, spray the tilapia fillets with the oil and then season with the salt, lemon pepper, and OLD BAY® seasoning until evenly coated. Open the

fryer, add the tilapia in it, close it and cook for 7 minutes, or until nicely golden and cooked, turning the fillets halfway through the frying. When Air Fry Oven beeps, open its lid, transfer tilapia fillets onto a serving plate and serve.

Nutrition:
- Calories: 36
- Fats: 0.75 g
- Protein: 7.4 g

Tomato Basil Scallops

Preparation Time: 5 minutes
Cooking Time: 15 minutes
Servings: 2
Ingredients:
- 8 jumbo sea scallops, wild-caught
- 1 tbsp. tomato paste
- 12 lb. frozen spinach, thawed and dried out
- 1 tbsp. fresh basil, chopped
- 1 tsp. ground black pepper
- 1 tsp. minced garlic
- 1 tsp. salt
- ¾ cup heavy whipping cream, reduced fat

Directions:
1. Switch the Air Fry Oven on, insert the basket, grease it with olive oil, close it and set it at 350ºF.
2. Meanwhile, take a 7-inch baking pan, grease it with oil and place the spinach in it in an even layer.
3. Spray the scallops with oil, sprinkle with ½ tsp. each of salt and black pepper and then place the scallops over the spinach.
4. Place the tomato paste in a bowl, whisk in the cream, basil, garlic, and remaining salt and black pepper until smooth, and then pour over the scallops.
5. Open the fryer, place the pan in it, close it and cook for 10 minutes, or until thoroughly cooked and hot.
6. Serve straight away.

Nutrition:
- Calories: 359
- Carbs: 6 g
- Fats: 33 g
- Protein: 9 g

Shrimp Scampi

Preparation Time: 5 minutes
Cooking Time: 12 minutes
Servings: 4
Ingredients:
- 1 lb. shrimp, peeled, deveined
- 1 tbsp. minced garlic
- 1 tbsp. minced basil
- 1 tbsp. lemon juice
- 1 tsp. dried chives
- 1 tsp. dried basil
- 2 tsp. red pepper flakes
- 4 tbsp. butter, unsalted
- 2 tbsp. chicken stock

Directions:
1. Switch the Air Fry Oven on, insert the basket, grease it with olive oil, close it and set it at 350ºF.
2. Add the butter in it along with the red pepper and garlic and cook for 2 minutes or until the butter has melted.
3. Then add the remaining ingredients in the pan, stir until mixed and continue cooking for 5 minutes, or until shrimps have cooked, stirring halfway through.
4. When done, remove the pan from the Air Fry Oven, stir the shrimp scampi, let it rest for 1 minute and then stir again.
5. Garnish the shrimps with the basil leaves and serve.

Nutrition:
- Calories: 221
- Carbs: 1 g
- Fats: 13 g
- Protein: 23 g

Salmon Cakes

Preparation Time: 5 minutes
Cooking Time: 12 minutes
Servings: 2
Ingredients:
- ½ cup almond flour
- 15 oz. cooked pink salmon
- ¼ tsp. ground black pepper
- 2 tsp. Dijon mustard
- 2 tbsp. chopped fresh dill
- 2 tbsp. mayonnaise, reduced fat
- 1 egg, pastured
- 2 lemon wedges

Directions:
1. Switch the Air Fry Oven on, insert the basket, grease it with olive oil, close it and set it at 350ºF.
2. Meanwhile, place all the ingredients in a bowl, except for the lemon wedges, stir until combined and then shape into four patties, each about 4 inches. Open the fryer, add the salmon patties in it, spray oil over them, close it and cook for 12 minutes or until nicely golden and crispy, flipping the patties halfway through the frying.

3.   When Air Fry Oven beeps, open its lid, transfer salmon patties onto a serving plate and serve.

Nutrition:
- Calories: 517
- Carbs: 15 g
- Fats: 27 g
- Protein: 52 g

Cilantro Lime Shrimps

Preparation Time: 25 minutes
Cooking Time: 21 minutes
Servings: 4
Ingredients:
- ½-lb. shrimp, peeled, deveined
- ½ tsp. minced garlic
- 1 tbsp. cilantro, chopped
- ½ tsp. paprika
- ¾ tsp. salt
- ½ tsp. ground cumin
- 2 tbsp. lemon juice

Directions:
1.   Take 6 wooden skewers and let them soak in warm water for 20 minutes
2.   Meanwhile, switch the Air Fry Oven on, insert the basket, grease it with olive oil, close it and set it at 350ºF.
3.   Whisk together the lemon juice, paprika, salt, cumin, and garlic in a large bowl, then add the shrimps and toss until well coated.
4.   Dry out the skewers and then thread the shrimps in them.
5.   Open the fryer, add the shrimps in it in a single layer, spray oil over them, close it and cook for 8 minutes or until nicely golden and cooked, turning the skewers halfway through the frying.
6.   When Air Fry Oven beeps, open it, transfer shrimps onto a serving plate and keep them warm.
7.   Cook the remaining shrimp skewers in the same manner and serve.

Nutrition:
- Calories: 59
- Carbs: 0.3 g
- Fats: 1.5 g
- Protein: 11 g

Cajun Style Shrimp

Preparation Time: 3 minutes
Cooking Time: 10 minutes
Servings: 2
Ingredients:
- ⅛ oz. salt
- 1/16 oz. smoked paprika
- 1/16 oz. garlic powder
- 1/16 oz. Italian seasoning
- 1/16 oz. chili powder
- ⅓2 oz. onion powder
- ⅓2 oz. cayenne pepper
- ⅓2 oz. black pepper
- ⅓2 oz. dried thyme
- 1 lb. large shrimp, peeled and unveiled
- 2 tbsp. olive oil
- Lime wedges, for serving

Directions:
1.   Select "Preheat" in the Air Fry Oven, set the temperature to 190°C and press "Start/Pause." Combine all the seasonings in a large bowl. Set aside
2.   Mix the shrimp with the olive oil until they are evenly coated. Sprinkle the dressing mixture over the shrimp and stir until well coated. Place the shrimp in the preheated Air Fry Oven.
3.   Select the Shrimp set the time to 5 minutes and press "Start/Pause." Shake the baskets in the middle of cooking. Serve with lime wedges.

Nutrition:
- Calories: 126
- Fats: 6 g
- Carbs: 2 g
- Protein: 33 g

CHAPTER 4: DINNER

Crispy Salt and Pepper Tofu

Preparation Time: 5 minutes

Cooking Time: 15 minutes

Servings: 4

Ingredients:

- ¼ cup chickpea flour
- ¼ cup arrowroot (or cornstarch)
- 1 tsp. sea salt
- 1 tsp. granulated garlic
- ½ tsp. freshly grated black pepper
- 1 (15-oz.) package tofu, firm or extra-firm
- Cooking oil spray (sunflower, safflower, or refined coconut)
- Asian Spicy Sweet Sauce, optional

Directions:

1. In a medium bowl, combine the flour, arrowroot, salt, garlic, and pepper. Stir well to combine.
2. Cut the tofu into cubes (no need to press—if it's a bit watery, that's fine!). Place the cubes into the flour mixture. Toss well to coat. Spray the tofu with oil and toss again. (The spray will help the coating better stick to the tofu.)
3. Spray the air fry basket with the oil. Place the tofu in a single layer in the air fry basket (you may have to do this in 2 batches, depending on the size of your appliance) and spray the tops with oil. Fry for 8 minutes. Remove the air fry basket and spray again with oil. Toss gently or turn the pieces over. Spray with oil again and fry for another 7 minutes, or until golden-browned and very crisp.
4. Serve immediately, either plain or with the Asian Spicy Sweet Sauce.

Nutrition:

- Calories: 148
- Total Fats: 5 g
- Sodium: 473 mg
- Carbs: 14 g Fiber: 1 g
- Protein: 11 g

Air Fryer Chicken Wings

Preparation Time: 5 minutes

Cooking Time: 20 minutes

Servings: 4

Ingredients:

- 4 Chicken wings
- ½ tsp. Sea salt
- ½ tsp. Black pepper
- 1 oz. Smoked paprika
- ½ tsp. Garlic powder
- ½ tsp. Onion powder
- ½ tsp. Baking powder
- 2 tbsp. Olive oil

Directions:

1. Take the chicken wing out of the refrigerator and pat them dry (if you remove as much moisture as possible, you will get a crispy wing skin).
2. Mix the sea salt, black pepper, smoked paprika, garlic powder, onion powder and baking powder in a small bowl or baking dish.
3. Sprinkle the spice mixture on the wings and throw it to cover.
4. Place the wings on the respective basket. In Ninja Foodie this is known as the "Cook&Crisp" basket.
5. Drizzle the chicken wings with olive oil.
6. Use the "Air Crisp" setting at 400°F on the Air Fry Oven to cook the wings for 14 minutes on each side.
7. Enjoy hot wings!

Nutrition:

- Calories: 32
- Protein: 2 g
- Fats: 1.73 g
- Carbs: 2.56 g

Spicy Parmesan Chicken Wings

Preparation Time: 5 minutes

Cooking Time: 35 minutes

Servings: 5

Ingredients:

- 2 Chicken wings
- ½ tsp. Sea salt
- ½ tsp. Black pepper
- 2 Bell pepper
- ½ tsp. Garlic powder
- ½ tsp. Onion powder
- ½ tsp. Baking powder
- 1 lb. Parmesan cheese

Directions:

1. Take the chicken wing out of the refrigerator and pat them dry.
2. Mix sea salt, black pepper, bell pepper, garlic powder, onion powder and baking powder in a small bowl.
3. Sprinkle some of the spice mixture on the wings and throw it to cover.
4. Place the wings on a flat layer in the Air Fry Oven.
5. Place the chicken in the Air Fry Oven at 400°F and cook for 30 minutes. To make the wings crispy quickly, you have to turn them about halfway.
6. Serve the chicken wings with the rest of the spicy parmesan sauce.

Nutrition:
- Calories: 176
- Protein: 2.02 g
- Fats: 15.19 g
- Carbs: 9.79 g

Buffalo Cauliflower Bites

Preparation Time: 5 minutes
Cooking Time: 25 minutes
Servings: 4
Ingredients:
- 2 lb. Cauliflower
- 2 Garlic cloves
- 3 tbsp Oil
- ½ tsp. Salt
- 1 lb. Blue cheese
- For the Buffalo Sauce:
- 1 lb. Hot Sauce
- 1 tbsp Butter
- 1 lb. Worcestershire sauce

Directions:
1. Cut the cauliflower into florets of equal size and place in a large bowl.
2. Cut each clove of garlic into 3 pieces and smash them with the side of your knife. Don't be afraid to smash the garlic. You want to expose as much of the garlic surface as possible so that it cooks well. Add this to the cauliflower.
3. Pour over the oil and add salt. Mix well until the cauliflower is well covered with oil and salt.
4. Turn on the Air Fry Oven at 400°F for 20 minutes and add the cauliflower. Turn it in half once.

To make the Sauce, whisk the hot sauce, butter and Worcestershire sauce in a small bowl.

5. Once the cauliflower is cooked, place it in a large bowl. Pour the hot sauce over the cauliflower and mix well.
6. Put the cauliflower back in the Air Fry Oven. Set it to 400F for 3-4 minutes so the sauce becomes a little firm.
7. Serve with the blue cheese.

Nutrition:
- Calories: 69
- Protein: 1.87 g
- Fats: 6.06 g
- Carbs: 1.99 g

Spicy Dry-Rubbed Chicken Wings

Preparation Time: 5 minutes
Cooking Time: 45 minutes
Servings: 6
Ingredients:
- 2 Chicken wings
- ¼ cup Spicy dry massage

Directions:
1. Take the chicken out of the fridge and let it approach room temperature (30 minutes). Preheat the oven to 400°F.
2. Place the chicken in a Ziploc® bag with the spicy dry massage.
3. Shake the bag so that the mixture covers the chicken evenly.
1. Store in the refrigerator for at least 4 hours, ideally overnight.

Nutrition:
- Calories: 230
- Protein: 31.02 g
- Fats: 11.54 g
- Carbs: 1.11 g

Air Fryer Steak Bites and Mushrooms

Preparation Time: 5 minutes
Cooking Time: 25 minutes
Servings: 4
Ingredients:
- 1 lb. Beef cut into cubes
- 3 tbsp Olive oil
- ½ tbsp Montreal steak seasoning
- 2 Mushrooms

Directions:

1. Preheat the empty air fryer to 390 ° F with a crisp plate or basket for 4 minutes.

2. Pat the meat dry. As the Air Fry Oven heats up, throw beef cubes with olive oil and Montreal spices.

3. Halve the mushrooms. Put the beef cubes and halved mushrooms into the preheated Air Fry Oven and gently shake to combine.

4. Set the Air Fry Oven temperature to 390°F and the timer to 8 minutes.

5. Stop after 3 minutes and shake the basket. Repeat this process every 2 minutes, or until the beef cubes have reached the desired degree of cooking. Lift a large piece out and test it with a meat thermometer or cut and look in the middle to see the progress. Note that the meat will continue to cook as soon as it is removed from the Air Fry Oven and resting.

6. Let the meat rest for a few minutes before serving and then enjoy.

Nutrition:

- Calories: 583
- Protein: 32.38 g
- Fats: 27.25 g
- Carbs: 61.98 g

Pecan Crusted Chicken

Preparation Time: 10 minutes
Cooking Time: 25 minutes
Servings: 6
Ingredients:

- 2 lb. Chicken tenders
- ½ tsp. Salt
- ½ tsp. Pepper
- 1 Smoked paprika
- 1 tbsp Honey
- 1 lb. Mustard
- 1 lb. Pecans, finely chopped

Directions:

1. Place the chicken tenders in a large bowl.

2. Add the salt, pepper and smoked paprika and mix well until the chicken is covered with the spices.

3. Pour in the honey and mustard and mix well.

4. Place the finely chopped pecans on a plate.

5. Roll the tenders into the shredded pecans, one chicken tender at a time, until both sides are covered. Brush off excess material.

6. Place the chicken tenders in the air fry basket and continue until all the tenders have been coated and are in the air fry basket.

7. Set the Air Fry Oven to 350°F for 12 minutes until the chicken is cooked through and the pecans are golden brown before serving.

Nutrition:

- Calories: 95
- Protein: 3.08 g
- Fats: 8.18 g
- Carbs: 3.16 g

Chicken Tikka Kebab

Preparation Time: 10 minutes
Cooking Time: 30 minutes
Servings: 6
Ingredients:

- 2 lb. Chicken
- 1 lb. Marinade
- 2 tbsp Oil
- 2 Onions
- 2 Green Pepper
- 2 Red Pepper

Directions:

1. Add the chicken and spread the marinade on each side. Let it rest in the fridge for between 30 minutes and 8 hours.

2. Add the oil, onions, green and red peppers to the marinade for cooking. Mix well.

3. Thread the marinated chicken, peppers and onions into the skewers in between.

4. Lightly, grease the air fry basket.

5. Arrange the chicken sticks in the Air Fry Oven. Cook them at 356°F for 10 minutes.

6. Turn the chicken sticks and cook for another 7 minutes, then serve.

Nutrition:

- Calories: 147
- Protein: 10.25 g
- Fats: 10.68 g
- Carbs: 1.85 g

Air Fryer Brussels sprouts

Preparation Time: 10 minutes

Cooking Time: 15 minutes

Servings: 2

Ingredients:

- ¼ c. balsamic vinegar
- 3 tbsp. extra-virgin olive oil
- ½ tsp. Kosher salt
- ½ tsp. Freshly ground black pepper

Directions:

1. Remove the hard ends of the Brussels sprouts and remove any damaged outer leaves. Rinse them under cold water and pat dry. If the sprouts are large, cut them in half. Add the oil, salt and pepper.

2. Arrange the Brussels sprouts in a single layer in your Air Fry Oven and work in batches if not all fit. Cook for 8–12 minutes at 374°F and shake the pan halfway through the cooking process to brown it evenly. They are done when they are lightly browned and crispy at the edges.

3. Serve the sprouts warm, optionally with balsamic reduction and parmesan.

Nutrition:

- Calories: 1197
- Protein: 125.58 g
- Fats: 65.97 g
- Carbs: 16.97 g

Crispy Air Fried Tofu

Preparation Time: 10 minutes

Cooking Time: 50 minutes

Servings: 8

Ingredients:

- 2 c. almond flour
- ½ tsp. baking soda
- ¼ tsp. kosher salt
- ¼ c. butter, room temperature
- ¼ c. almond butter
- 3 tbsp. honey
- 1 large egg
- 1 tsp. pure vanilla extract
- 1 c. semisweet chocolate chips
- ½ tsp. Flaky sea salt
- 1 lb. Tofu

Directions:

1. Squeeze the tofu for at least 15 minutes by placing either a heavy pan or a pan on top and letting the moisture drain. When you're done, cut the tofu into bite-sized blocks and put it in a bowl.

2. Mix all the remaining ingredients in a small bowl. Drizzle over the tofu and toss to cover. Let the tofu marinate for another 15 minutes.

3. Preheat your air fryer to 374°F. Add the tofu blocks to your air fry basket in a single layer. Let cook for 10–15 minutes and shake the pan occasionally for an even cooking.

Nutrition:

- Calories: 247
- Protein: 3.83 g
- Fats: 18.05 g
- Carbs: 21.99 g

Buttermilk Fried Mushrooms

Preparation Time: 5 minutes

Cooking Time: 30 minutes

Servings: 2

Ingredients:

- 2 tbsp. olive oil
- 1 tsp. kosher salt
- 1 tsp. cayenne
- 1 tsp. paprika
- 1 tsp. garlic powder
- 1 tsp. onion powder
- 1 tsp. oregano
- 2 lemons, sliced thinly crosswise
- 2 lb. Mushrooms
- 1 lb. Buttermilk
- 2 cups Flour

Directions:

1. Preheat the Air Fry Oven to 374°C. Clean the mushrooms and place them in a large bowl with buttermilk. Let marinate for 15 minutes.

2. Mix the flour and spices in a large bowl. Put the mushrooms out of the buttermilk (keep the buttermilk). Dip each mushroom in the flour mixture, shake off any excess flour, dip again in the buttermilk and then again in the flour.

1. Grease the bottom of your air pan well and place the mushrooms in a layer, leaving space between the mushrooms. Let it cook for 5 minutes, then roughly coat all sides with a little oil to promote browning. Cook for another 5–10 minutes until golden brown and crispy.

Nutrition:

- Calories: 380
- Protein: 49.65 g

- Fats: 18.15 g
- Carbs: 6.86 g

Crispy Baked Avocado Tacos

Preparation Time: 10 minutes
Cooking Time: 20 minutes
Servings: 5
Ingredients:
- 2 Avocado
- 1 cup Flour
- 1 Panko

For the Sauce:
- 6 slices of ham (we used Applegate brand)
- 4 eggs
- ¼ cup full-fat coconut milk
- ¼ cup orange bell peppers, chopped
- ¼ cup red bell peppers, chopped
- ¼ cup yellow onions, chopped
- ½ tsp. Salt & pepper, to taste
- 1 tbsp Olive oil or coconut oil to sauté veggies

Directions:
1. Combine all the salsa ingredients and put them in the fridge.
2. Halve the avocado lengthwise and remove the pit. Lay the avocado skin-face down and cut each half into 4 equal pieces. Then gently peel off the skin.
3. Preheat the oven to 446°C or the Air Fry Oven to 374°F. Arrange your work area so that you have a bowl of flour, a bowl of sauce, a bowl of panko with salt and pepper, and a baking sheet lined with parchment at the end.
4. Dip each avocado slice first in the flour, then in the sauce and then in the panko. Place on the prepared baking sheet and bake for 10 minutes or fry in the air. Lightly brown after half of the cooking process.
5. While cooking avocados, combine all the ingredients in the bowls.
6. Pour some mixture on each tortilla, top with 2 pieces of avocado and drizzle with sauce. Serve immediately and enjoy!

Nutrition:
- Calories: 193
- Protein: 13.7 g
- Fats: 13.25 g
- Carbs: 4.69 g

Chicken Cordon Bleu

Preparation Time: 60 minutes
Cooking Time: 40 minutes
Servings: 6
Ingredients:
- 1 garlic clove
- 2 eggs
- 2 tsp. butter, melted
- 1 cup bread, ground
- ¼ cup flour
- 2 tsp. fresh thyme
- 16 slices Swiss cheese
- 8 slices ham
- 4 chicken breasts

Directions:
1. Preheat the Air Fry Oven to 350ºF.
2. Flatten out the chicken breasts and then fill them with 2 cheese slices, 2 ham slices, and then cheese again.
3. Roll the chicken breasts, using a toothpick to keep them together.
4. Mix the garlic, thyme, and bread together with the butter. Beat the eggs and season the flour with pepper and salt.
5. Pass the chicken rolls through the flour, then the eggs, and then the breadcrumbs. Add to the Air Fry Oven to cook.
- After 20 minutes, take the chicken rolls out and them cool down before serving.

Nutrition:
- Calories: 387
- Carbs: 18 g
- Fats: 20 g
- Protein: 33 g

Fried Chicken

Preparation Time: 20 minutes
Cooking Time: 25 minutes
Servings: 4
Ingredients:
- 1 lemon
- 1 ginger, grated
- ½ tsp. Ground pepper, salt, and garlic powder
- 1 lb. chopped chicken
- 1 tbsp Oil

Directions:

1.   Add the chicken to a bowl with the rest of the ingredients. Let it set for a bit to marinate.

2.   After 15 minutes, add some oil to the Air Fry Oven and let it heat up to 320°F.

3.   Place the chicken in the Air Fry Oven to cook for 25 minutes, shaking it a few times to cook through. Serve warm.

Nutrition:

- Calories: 345
- Carbs: 23 g
- Fats: 3 g
- Protein: 3 g

Seasoned Tomatoes

Preparation Time: 10 minutes

Cooking Time: 10 minutes

Servings: 2

Ingredients:

- 3 tomatoes, halved
- Olive oil cooking spray
- Salt and ground black pepper
- 1 tbsp. fresh basil, chopped

Directions:

1.   Drizzle the tomatoes halves with the olive oil.

2.   Sprinkle with salt, black pepper and basil.

3.   Press the "Power" button of the Air Fry Oven and turn the dial to select the "Air Fry" mode.

4.   Press the "Time" button and again turn the dial to set the cooking time to 10 minutes.

5.   Now push the "Temp" button and rotate the dial to set the temperature at 320°F.

6.   Press the "Start/Pause" button to start.

7.   Open the unit when it has reached the temperature, when it beeps.

8.   Arrange the tomatoes in the air fry basket and insert them in the oven.

9.   Serve warm.

Nutrition:

- Calories: 34
- Fats: 0.4 g
- Carbs: 7.2 g
- Protein: 1.7 g

Filled Tomatoes

Preparation Time: 15 minutes

Cooking Time: 15 minutes

Servings: 4

Ingredients:

- 2 large tomatoes
- ½ cup broccoli, chopped finely
- ½ cup Cheddar cheese, shredded
- Salt and ground black pepper
- ½ tsp. dried thyme, crushed

Directions:

1.   Carefully, cut the top of each tomato d scoop out the pulp and seeds.

2.   In a bowl, mix together the chopped broccoli, cheese, salt and black pepper.

3.   Stuff each tomato with the broccoli mixture evenly.

4.   Press the "Power" button of the Air Fry Oven and turn the dial to select the "Air Fry" mode.

5.   Press the "Time" button and again turn the dial to set the cooking time to 15 minutes.

6.   Now push the "Temp" button and rotate the dial to set the temperature at 355°F.

7.   Press the "Start/Pause" button to start.

8.   Open the unit when it has reached the temperature, when it beeps.

9.   Arrange the tomatoes in a basket and insert them in the Air Fry Oven.

10.   Serve warm with the garnishing of thyme.

Nutrition:

- Calories: 206
- Fats: 15.6 g
- Carbs: 9 g
- Protein: 9.4 g

Parmesan Asparagus

Preparation Time: 10 minutes

Cooking Time: 10 minutes

Servings: 3

Ingredients:

- 1 lb. fresh asparagus, trimmed
- 1 tbsp. Parmesan cheese, grated
- 1 tbsp. butter, melted
- 1 tsp. garlic powder
- Salt and ground black pepper

Directions:

1.   In a bowl, mix together the asparagus, cheese, butter, garlic powder, salt, and black pepper.

2. Press the "Power" button of the Air Fry Oven and turn the dial to select the "Air Fry" mode.

3. Press the "Time" button and again turn the dial to set the cooking time to 10 minutes.

4. Now push the "Temp" button and rotate the dial to set the temperature at 400°F.

5. Press the "Start/Pause" button to start.

6. Open the unit when it has reached the temperature, when it beeps.

7. Arrange the veggie mixture in a basket and insert them in the Air Fry Oven.

8. Serve hot.

Nutrition:
- Calories: 73
- Fats: 4.4 g
- Carbs: 6.6 g
- Protein: 4.2 g

Almond Asparagus

Preparation Time: 15 minutes
Cooking Time: 16 minutes
Servings: 3
Ingredients:
- 1 lb. asparagus
- 2 tbsp. olive oil
- 2 tbsp. balsamic vinegar
- Salt and ground black pepper

Directions:
1. In a bowl, mix together the asparagus, oil, vinegar, salt, and black pepper.

2. Press the "Power" button of the Air Fry Oven and turn the dial to select the "Air Fry" mode.

3. Press the "Time" button and again turn the dial to set the cooking time to 6 minutes.

4. Now push the "Temp" button and rotate the dial to set the temperature at 400°F.

5. Press the "Start/Pause" button to start.

6. Open the unit when it has reached the temperature, when it beeps.

7. Arrange the veggie mixture in a basket and insert them in the Air Fry Oven.

8. Serve hot.

Nutrition:
- Calories: 173
- Fats: 14.8 g
- Carbs: 8.2 g
- Protein: 5.6 g

Spicy Butternut Squash

Preparation Time: 15 minutes
Cooking Time: 20 minutes
Servings: 4
Ingredients:
- 1 medium butternut squash, peeled, seeded and cut into chunks
- 2 tsp. cumin seeds
- ⅛ tsp. garlic powder
- ⅛ tsp. chili flakes, crushed
- Salt and ground black pepper
- 1 tbsp. olive oil
- 2 tbsp. pine nuts
- 2 tbsp. fresh cilantro, chopped

Directions:
1. In a bowl, mix together the squash, spices, and oil.

2. Press the "Power" button of the Air Fry Oven and turn the dial to select the "Air Fry" mode.

3. Press the "Time" button and again turn the dial to set the cooking time to 20 minutes.

4. Now push the "Temp" button and rotate the dial to set the temperature at 375°F.

5. Press the "Start/Pause" button to start.

6. Open the unit when it has reached the temperature, when it beeps.

7. Arrange the squash chunks in a basket and insert them in the Air Fry Oven.

8. Serve hot with the garnishing of pine nuts and cilantro.

Nutrition:
- Calories: 191
- Fats: 7 g
- Carbs: 34.3 g
- Protein: 3.7 g

Sweet & Spicy Parsnips

Preparation Time: 15 minutes
Cooking Time: 44 minutes
Servings: 5
Ingredients:
- 1 ½ lb. parsnip, peeled and cut into 1-inch chunks
- 1 tbsp. butter, melted
- 2 tbsp. honey
- 1 tbsp. dried parsley flakes, crushed

- ¼ tsp. red pepper flakes, crushed
- Salt and ground black pepper

Directions:

1. In a large bowl, mix together the parsnips and butter.
2. Press the "Power" button of the Air Fry Oven and turn the dial to select the "Air Fry" mode.
3. Press the "Time" button and again turn the dial to set the cooking time to 44 minutes.
4. Now push the "Temp" button and rotate the dial to set the temperature at 355°F.
5. Press the "Start/Pause" button to start.
6. Open the unit when it has reached the temperature, when it beeps.
7. Arrange the squash chunks in a basket and insert them in the Air Fry Oven.
8. Meanwhile, in another large bowl, mix together the remaining ingredients.
9. After 40 minutes of cooking, press the "Start/Pause" button to pause the unit.
10. Transfer the parsnips chunks into the bowl of honey mixture and toss to coat well.
11. Again, arrange the parsnip chunks in the air fry basket and insert in the Air Fry Oven.
12. Serve hot.

Nutrition:

- Calories: 149
- Fats: 2.7 g
- Carbs: 31.5 g
- Protein: 1.7 g

Pesto Tomatoes

Preparation Time: 15 minutes
Cooking Time: 20 minutes
Servings: 4
Ingredients:

- 3 large heirloom tomatoes cut into ½ inch thick slices.
- 8 oz. feta cheese, cut into ½ inch thick slices.
- ½ cup red onions, thinly sliced
- 1 tbsp. olive oil

Directions:

1. Spread some pesto on each tomato slice. Top each tomato slice with a feta slice, onion and drizzle with oil.
2. Press the "Power" button of the Air Fry Oven and turn the dial to select the "Air Fry" mode.

Press the "Time" button and again turn the dial to set the cooking time to 14 minutes.

3. Now push the "Temp" button and rotate the dial to set the temperature at 390°F. Press the "Start/Pause" button to start.
4. Open the unit when it has reached the temperature, when it beeps. Arrange the tomatoes in a basket and insert them in the Air Fry Oven.
5. Serve warm.

Nutrition:

- Calories: 480
- Fats: 41.9 g
- Carbs: 13 g
- Protein: 15.4 g

Roasted Cauliflower with Nuts & Raisins

Preparation Time: 5 minutes
Cooking Time: 20 minutes
Servings: 4
Ingredients:

- 1 small cauliflower head, cut into florets
- 2 tbsp. pine nuts, toasted
- 2 tbsp. raisins soak in boiling water and dried
- 1 tsp. curry powder
- ½ tsp. sea salt
- 3 tbsp. olive oil

Directions:

1. Preheat your Air Fry Oven to 320°F for 2 minutes. Add all the ingredients to a bowl and toss to combine.
2. Add the cauliflower mixture to the air fry basket and cook for 15 minutes.

Nutrition:

- Calories: 264
- Fats: 26 g
- Carbs: 8 g
- Protein: 2 g

Spicy Herb Chicken Wings

Preparation Time: 15 minutes
Cooking Time: 15 minutes
Servings: 6
Ingredients:

- 4 lbs. chicken wings
- ½ tbsp. ginger
- 2 tbsp. vinegar

- 1 fresh lime juice
- 1 tbsp. olive oil
- 2 tbsp. soy sauce
- 6 garlic cloves, minced
- 1 habanero, chopped
- ¼ tsp. cinnamon
- ½ tsp. sea salt

Directions:
1. Preheat your Air Fry Oven to 390°F.
2. Add all the ingredients except the chicken to a large bowl and combine well.
3. Place the chicken wings into the marinade mix and store in the fridge for 2 hours.
4. Add the chicken wings to the Air Fry Oven and cook for 15 minutes. Serve hot!

Nutrition:
- Calories: 673
- Fats: 29 g
- Carbs: 9 g
- Protein: 39 g

Lamb Meatballs

Preparation Time: 5 minutes
Cooking Time: 15 minutes
Servings: 4
Ingredients:
- 1 lb. ground lamb
- 1 egg white
- ½ tsp. sea salt
- 2 tbsp. parsley, fresh, chopped
- 1 tbsp. coriander, chopped
- 2 garlic cloves, minced
- 1 tbsp. olive oil
- 1 tbsp. mint, chopped

Directions:
1. Preheat your Air Fry Oven to 320°F.
2. Add all the ingredients in a mixing bowl and combine well.
3. Form small meatballs from the mixture and place them in air fry basket and cook for 15 minutes. Serve hot!

Nutrition:
- Calories: 312
- Fats: 9.8 g
- Carbs: 12.3 g
- Protein: 23 g

Sweet & Sour Chicken Skewer

Preparation Time: 5 minutes
Cooking Time: 18 minutes
Servings: 4
Ingredients:
- 1 lb. chicken tenders
- ¼ tsp. pepper
- 4 garlic cloves, minced
- 1 ½ tbsp. soy sauce
- 2 tbsp. pineapple juice
- 1 tbsp. sesame oil
- ½ tsp. ginger, minced

Directions:
1. Preheat your Air Fry Oven to 390°F.
2. Combine all the ingredients in a bowl, except for the chicken.
3. Skewer the chicken tenders, them then soak them in the marinade for 2 hours.
4. Add tenders to the Air Fry Oven and cook for 18 minutes. Serve hot!

Nutrition:
- Calories: 217
- Fats: 3 g
- Carbs: 15.3 g
- Protein: 21.3 g

Green Stuffed Peppers

Preparation Time: 5 minutes
Cooking Time: 25 minutes
Servings: 3
Ingredients:
- 3 green bell peppers, tops and seeds removed
- 1 onion, medium-sized, diced
- 1 carrot, thinly diced
- 1 small cauliflower, shredded
- 1 tsp. garlic powder
- 1 tsp. coriander
- 1 tsp. mixed spices
- 1 tsp. Chinese five spice
- 1 tbsp. olive oil
- 3 tbsp. any soft cheese
- 1 zucchini, thinly diced
- ¼ yellow pepper, thinly diced

Directions:

1. Sauté the onion with the olive oil in a wok over medium heat.
2. Add the cauliflower and seasonings. Cook for 5 minutes, stirring to combine.
3. Add the vegetables (carrot, zucchini, yellow pepper) and cook for an additional 5 minutes more.
4. Fill each of the green peppers with 1 tbsp. of soft cheese.
5. Then stuff them with cauliflower mixture.
6. Cap the stuffed peppers with the pepper tops and cook in the Air Fry Oven for 15 minutes at 390°F.

Nutrition:
- Calories: 272
- Fats: 12.7 g
- Carbs: 26 g
- Protein: 17 g

Beef Meatballs in Tomato Sauce

Preparation Time: 5 minutes
Cooking Time: 12 minutes
Servings: 3
Ingredients:
- 11 oz. minced beef
- 1 onion, chopped finely
- 1 tbsp. fresh parsley, chopped
- 1 cup tomato sauce
- 1 egg
- Salt and pepper to taste
- 1 tbsp. fresh thyme, chopped

Directions:
1. Mix all the ingredients in a mixing bowl, except the tomato sauce. Form 11 meatballs with the mixture. Preheat your Air Fry Oven to 390°F.
2. Add the meatballs to the air fry basket and cook for 7 minutes. Transfer the meatballs to an oven-safe dish and pour the tomato sauce over them.
3. Put the dish in the air fry basket and cook for an additional 5 minute at 320°F.

Nutrition:
- Calories: 275
- Fats: 16 g
- Carbs: 2 g
- Protein: 20 g

Mustard Pork Balls

Preparation Time: 5 minutes

Cooking Time: 15 minutes
Servings: 4
Ingredients:
- 7 oz. minced pork
- 1 tsp. organic honey
- 1 tsp. Dijon mustard
- 1 tbsp. cheddar cheese, grated
- ⅓ cup onion, diced
- Salt and pepper to taste
- A handful of fresh basil, chopped
- 1 tsp. garlic purée

Directions:
1. In a bowl, mix the meat with all of the seasonings and form balls.
2. Place the pork balls into the Air Fry Oven and cook for 15 minutes at 392°F.

Nutrition:
- Calories: 121
- Fats: 6.8 g
- Carbs: 2.7 g
- Protein: 11.3 g

Garlic Pork Chops

Preparation Time: 5 minutes
Cooking Time: 16 minutes
Servings: 4
Ingredients:
- 4 pork chops
- 1 tbsp. coconut butter
- 2 tsp. minced garlic cloves
- 1 tbsp. coconut butter
- 2 tsp. parsley, chopped
- Salt and pepper to taste

Directions:
1. Preheat your air fryer to 350°F.
2. In a bowl, mix the coconut oil, seasonings, and butter. Coat the pork chops with this mixture.
3. Place the chops on the grill pan of your Air Fry oven cook them for 8 minutes per side.

Nutrition:
- Calories: 356
- Fats: 30 g
- Carbs: 2.3 g
- Protein: 19 g

Honey Ginger Salmon Fillets

Preparation Time: 5 minutes

Cooking Time: 10 minutes

Servings: 2

Ingredients:

- 2 salmon fillets
- 2 tbsp. fresh ginger, minced
- 2 garlic cloves, minced
- ¼ cup honey
- ⅓ cup orange juice
- ⅓ cup soy sauce
- 1 lemon, sliced

Directions:

1. Mix all the ingredients in a bowl.
2. Marinate the salmon fillets in the sauce for 2 hours in the fridge.
3. Add the marinated salmon to the air fry basket and cook at 395°F for 10 minutes. Garnish with fresh ginger and lemon slices.

Nutrition:

- Calories: 514
- Fats: 22 g
- Carbs: 39.5 g
- Protein: 41 g

Rosemary & Lemon Salmon

Preparation Time: 5 minutes

Cooking Time: 10 minutes

Servings: 2

Ingredients:

- 2 salmon fillets
- 1 dash pepper
- 2 lb. Fresh rosemary, chopped
- 2 slices of lemon

Directions:

1. Rub the rosemary over the salmon fillets, then season them with salt and pepper, and place lemon slices on top of salmon fillets.
2. Place in the fridge for 2 hours.
3. Preheat your Air Fry Oven to 320°F. Cook for 10 minutes.

Nutrition:

- Calories: 363
- Fats: 22 g
- Carbs: 8 g
- Protein: 40 g

Fish with Capers & Herb Sauce

Preparation Time: 5 minutes

Cooking Time: 15 minutes

Servings: 4

Ingredients:

- 2 cod fillets
- ¼ cup almond flour
- 1 tsp. Dijon Mustard
- 1 egg

For the Sauce:

- 2 tbsp. light sour cream
- 2 tsp. capers
- 1 tbsp. tarragon, chopped
- 1 tbsp. fresh dill, chopped
- 2 tbsp. red onion, chopped
- 2 tbsp. dill pickle, chopped

Directions:

1. Add all of the sauce ingredients into a small mixing bowl and mix until well blended then place in the fridge.
2. In a bowl, mix the Dijon mustard and the egg and sprinkle the flour over a plate.
3. Dip the cod fillets first in the egg mixture to coat, and then dip them into the flour, coating them on both sides.
4. Preheat your Air Fry Oven to 300°F, place the fillets into the Air Fry Oven and cook for 10 minutes.
5. Place the fillets on the serving dishes, drizzle with the sauce and serve.

Nutrition:

- Calories: 198
- Fats: 9.4 g
- Carbs: 17.6 g
- Protein: 11 g

Lemon Halibut

Preparation Time: 5 minutes

Cooking Time: 20 minutes

Servings: 4

Ingredients:

- 4 halibut fillets
- 1 egg, beaten
- 1 lemon, sliced
- ½ tsp. Salt and pepper to taste
- 1 tbsp. parsley, chopped

Directions:

1. Sprinkle the lemon juice over the halibut fillets.

2.   In a food processor mix the lemon slices, salt, pepper, and parsley.

3.   Take fillets and coat them with this mixture; then dip the fillets into the beaten egg.

4.   Cook the fillets in your Air Fry Oven at 350°F for 15 minutes.

Nutrition:
- Calories: 48
- Fats: 1 g
- Carbs: 2.5 g
- Protein: 9 g

Fried Cod & Spring Onion

Preparation Time: 5 minutes
Cooking Time: 20 minutes
Servings: 4
Ingredients:
- 7 oz. cod fillet, washed and dried
- 1 Spring onion, white and green parts, chopped
- A dash of sesame oil
- 5 tbsp. light soy sauce
- 1 tsp. dark soy sauce
- 3 tbsp. olive oil
- 5 slices of ginger
- 1 cup water
- ½ tsp. Salt and pepper to taste

Directions:
1.   Season the cod fillet with a dash of sesame oil, salt, and pepper. Preheat your Air Fry Oven to 356ºF. Cook the cod fillet in air fryer for 12 minutes.

2.   For the seasoning sauce, boil water in a pan along with both light and dark soy sauce on the stovetop and stir.

3.   In a small saucepan, heat the olive oil and add the ginger and white part of the spring onion. Fry until the ginger browns, then remove the ginger and onions.

4.   Top the cod fillet with shredded green onion. Pour the olive oil over the fillet and add the seasoning sauce on top.

Nutrition:
- Calories: 233
- Fats: 16 g
- Carbs: 15.5 g
- Protein: 6.7 g

CHAPTER 5: POULTRY

Herbed Cornish Game Hen

Preparation Time: 15 minutes
Cooking Time: 35 minutes
Servings: 4
Ingredients:

- 2 tbsp. avocado oil
- ½ tsp. dried oregano
- ½ tsp. dried rosemary
- ½ tsp. dried thyme
- ½ tsp. dried basil
- Salt and ground black pepper, as required
- 2 Cornish game hens

Directions:

1. In a bowl, mix together the oil, dried herbs, salt and black pepper.
2. Rub each hen with the herb mixture evenly.
3. Press the "Power" button of the Ninja Foodi Digital Air Fry Oven and turn the dial to select "Air Fry" mode.
4. Press the "Time" button and again turn the dial to set the cooking time to 35 minutes.
5. Now push the "Temp" button and rotate the dial to set the temperature at 360°F.
6. Press the "Start/Pause" button to start.
7. When the unit beeps to show that it is preheated, open the lid and grease the air fry basket.
8. Arrange the hens into the prepared basket breast-side down, and insert in the Air Fry Oven.
9. When the cooking time is completed, open the lid and transfer the hens onto a platter.
10. Cut each hen into pieces and serve.

Serving Suggestion: Serve alongside roasted veggies.
Variation Tip: You can use fresh herbs instead of dried herbs.
Nutrition:

- Calories: 895
- Fats: 62.9 g
- Saturated Fats: 17.4 g
- Carbs: 0.7 g
- Fiber: 0.5 g
- Protein: 75.9 g

Cajun Spiced Whole Chicken

Preparation Time: 15 minutes
Cooking Time: 1 hour 10 minutes
Servings: 6
Ingredients:

- ¼ cup butter, softened
- 2 tsp. dried rosemary
- 2 tsp. dried thyme
- 1 tbsp. Cajun seasoning
- 1 tbsp. onion powder
- 1 tbsp. garlic powder
- 1 tbsp. paprika
- 1 tsp. cayenne pepper
- Salt, as required
- 1 (3-lb.) whole chicken, neck and giblets removed

Directions:

1. In a bowl, add the butter, herbs, spices and salt and mix well.
2. Rub the chicken with spicy mixture generously.
3. With the help of kitchen twines, tie off the wings and legs.
4. Press the "Power" button of the Ninja Foodi Digital Air Fry Oven and turn the dial to select "Air Bake" mode.
5. Press the "Time" button and again turn the dial to set the cooking time to 70 minutes.
6. Now push the "Temp" button and rotate the dial to set the temperature at 380°F.
7. Press the "Start/Pause" button to start.
8. Open the unit when it has reached the temperature, when it beeps.
9. Arrange the chicken over the wire rack and insert them in the Air Fry Oven.
10. When the cooking time is completed, open the lid and place the chicken onto a platter for about 10 minutes before cutting.
11. Cut into desired sized pieces and serve.

Serving Suggestions: Serve alongside a fresh green salad.
Variation Tip: You can adjust the ratio of spices according to your choice.
Nutrition:

- Calories: 421
- Fats: 14.8 g
- Saturated Fats: 6.9 g

- Carbs: 2.3 g
- Fiber: 0.9 g
- Sugar: 0.5 g
- Protein: 66.3 g

Lemony Whole Chicken

Preparation Time: 15 minutes
Cooking Time: 1 hour 20 minutes
Servings: 8
Ingredients:
- 1 (5-lb.) whole chicken, neck and giblets removed
- Salt and ground black pepper, as required
- 2 fresh rosemary sprigs
- 1 small onion, peeled and quartered
- 1 garlic clove, peeled and cut in half
- 4 lemon zest slices
- 1 tbsp. extra-virgin olive oil
- 1 tbsp. fresh lemon juice

Directions:
1. Rub the inside and outside of chicken with salt and black pepper evenly.
2. Place the rosemary sprigs, onion quarters, garlic halves and lemon zest in the cavity of the chicken.
3. With the help of kitchen twines, tie off the wings and legs.
4. Arrange the chicken onto a greased baking pan and drizzle with the oil and lemon juice.
5. Press the "Power" button of the Ninja Foodi Digital Air Fry Oven and turn the dial to select "Air Bake" mode.
6. Press the "Time" button and again turn the dial to set the cooking time to 20 minutes.
7. Now push the "Temp" button and rotate the dial to set the temperature at 400°F.
8. Press the "Start/Pause" button to start.
9. Open the unit when it has reached the temperature, when it beeps.
10. Arrange the pan over the wire rack and insert them in the oven.
11. After 20 minutes of cooking, set the temperature to 375°F for 60 minutes.
12. When cooking time is completed, open the lid and place the chicken onto a platter for about 10 minutes before cutting.
13. Cut into desired piece sizes and serve.

Serving Suggestions: Serve alongside the steamed veggies.
Variation Tip: Lemon can be replaced with lime.
Nutrition:
- Calories: 448
- Fats: 10.4 g
- Saturated Fats: 2.7 g
- Carbs: 1 g
- Fiber: 0.4 g
- Sugar: 0.2 g
- Protein: 82 g

Crispy Chicken Legs

Preparation Time: 15 minutes
Cooking Time: 20 minutes
Servings: 3
Ingredients:
- 3 (8-oz.) chicken legs
- 1 cup buttermilk
- 2 cups white flour
- 1 tsp. garlic powder
- 1 tsp. onion powder
- 1 tsp. ground cumin
- 1 tsp. paprika
- Salt and ground black pepper, as required
- 1 tbsp. olive oil

Directions:
1. In a bowl, place the chicken legs and buttermilk and refrigerate for about 2 hours.
2. In a shallow dish, mix together the flour and the spices.
3. Remove the chicken from buttermilk.
4. Coat the chicken legs with flour mixture, then dip them into buttermilk and finally, coat with the flour mixture again.
5. Press the "Power" of the Ninja Foodi Digital Air Fry Oven and turn the dial to select "Air Fry" mode.
6. Press the "Time" button and again turn the dial to set the cooking time to 20 minutes.
7. Now push the "Temp" button and rotate the dial to set the temperature to 355°F.
8. Press the "Start/Pause" button to start.
9. When the unit beeps to show that it is preheated, open the lid and grease the air fry basket.
10. Arrange the chicken legs into the prepared air fry basket and drizzle with the oil.

11.   Insert the basket in the Air Fry Oven.

12.   When cooking time is completed, open the lid and serve hot.

Serving Suggestions: Serve with your favorite dip.

Variation Tip: White flour can be replaced with almond flour too.

Nutrition:

- Calories: 817
- Fats: 23.3 g
- Saturated Fats: 5.9 g
- Carbs: 69.5 g
- Fiber: 2.7 g
- Sugar: 4.7 g
- Protein: 77.4 g

Marinated Spicy Chicken Legs

Preparation Time: 10 minutes

Cooking Time: 20 minutes

Servings: 4

Ingredients:

- 4 chicken legs
- 3 tbsp. fresh lemon juice
- 3 tsp. ginger paste
- 3 tsp. garlic paste
- Salt, as required
- 4 tbsp. plain yogurt
- 2 tsp. red chili powder
- 1 tsp. ground cumin
- 1 tsp. ground coriander
- 1 tsp. ground turmeric
- Ground black pepper, as required

Directions:

1.   In a bowl, mix together the chicken legs, lemon juice, ginger, garlic and salt. Set aside for about 15 minutes.

2.   Meanwhile, in another bowl, mix together the yogurt and the spices.

3.   Add the chicken legs and coat with the spice mixture generously.

4.   Cover the bowl and refrigerate for at least 10–12 hours.

5.   Press the "Power" button of the Ninja Foodi Digital Air Fry Oven and turn the dial to select "Air Fry" mode.

6.   Press the "Time" button and again turn the dial to set the cooking time to 20 minutes.

7.   Now push the "Temp" button and rotate the dial to set the temperature to 440°F.

8.   Press the "Start/Pause" button to start.

9.   When the unit beeps to show that it is preheated, open the lid and grease the air fry basket.

10.   Place the chicken legs into the prepared air fry basket and insert them in the Air Fry Oven.

11.   When cooking time is completed, open the lid and serve hot.

Serving Suggestions: Serve with fresh greens.

Variation Tip: Lemon juice can be replaced with vinegar.

Nutrition:

- Calories: 461
- Fats: 17.6 g
- Saturated Fats: 5 g
- Carbs: 4.3 g
- Fiber: 0.9 g
- Sugar: 1.5 g
- Protein: 67.1 g

Gingered Chicken Drumsticks

Preparation Time: 10 minutes

Cooking Time: 25 minutes

Servings: 3

Ingredients:

- ¼ cup full-fat coconut milk
- 2 tsp. fresh ginger, minced
- 2 tsp. galangal, minced
- 2 tsp. ground turmeric
- Salt, as required
- 3 (6-oz.) chicken drumsticks

Directions:

1.   Place the coconut milk, galangal, ginger, and spices in a large bowl and mix well.

2.   Add the chicken drumsticks and coat with the marinade generously.

3.   Refrigerate to marinate for at least 6–8 hours.

4.   Press the "Power" button of the Ninja Foodi Digital Air Fry Oven and turn the dial to select "Air Fry" mode.

5.   Press the "Time" button and again turn the dial to set the cooking time to 25 minutes.

6.   Now push the "Temp" button and rotate the dial to set the temperature at 375°F.

7.   Press the "Start/Pause" button to start.

8. When the unit beeps to show that it is preheated, open the lid and grease the air fry basket.

9. Place the chicken drumsticks into the prepared air fry basket and insert them in the Air Fry Oven.

10. When the cooking time is completed, open the lid and serve hot.

Serving Suggestions: Serve alongside the lemony couscous.

Variation Tip: Coconut milk can be replaced with cream.

Nutrition:

- Calories: 347
- Fats: 14.8 g
- Saturated Fats: 6.9 g
- Carbs: 3.8 g
- Fiber: 1.1 g
- Sugar: 0.8 g
- Protein: 47.6 g

Crispy Chicken Drumsticks

Preparation Time: 15 minutes
Cooking Time: 25 minutes
Servings: 4
Ingredients:

- 4 chicken drumsticks
- 1 tbsp. adobo seasoning
- Salt, as required
- 1 tbsp. onion powder
- 1 tbsp. garlic powder
- ½ tbsp. paprika
- Ground black pepper, as required
- 2 eggs
- 2 tbsp. milk
- 1 cup all-purpose flour
- ¼ cup cornstarch

Directions:

1. Season the chicken drumsticks with the adobo seasoning and a pinch of salt.

2. Set aside for about 5 minutes.

3. In a small bowl, add the spices, salt and black pepper and mix well.

4. In a shallow bowl, add the eggs, milk and 1 tsp. of the spice mixture and beat until well combined.

5. In another shallow bowl, add the flour, cornstarch and the remaining spice mixture.

6. Coat the chicken drumsticks with the flour mixture and tap off excess.

7. Now, dip the chicken drumsticks in the egg mixture.

8. Again coat the chicken drumsticks with the flour mixture.

9. Arrange the chicken drumsticks onto a wire rack-lined baking sheet and set aside for about 15 minutes.

10. Now, arrange the chicken drumsticks onto a sheet pan and spray the chicken with cooking spray lightly.

11. Press the "Power" button of the Ninja Foodi Digital Air Fry Oven and turn the dial to select "Air Fry" mode.

12. Press the "Time" button and again turn the dial to set the cooking time to 25 minutes.

13. Now push the "Temp" button and rotate the dial to set the temperature at 350°F.

14. Press the "Start/Pause" button to start.

15. When the unit beeps to show that it is preheated, open the lid and grease the air fry basket.

16. Place the chicken drumsticks into the prepared air fry basket and insert them in the Air Fry Oven.

17. When the cooking time is completed, open the lid and serve hot.

Serving Suggestions: Serve with French fries.

Variation Tip: Make sure to coat chicken pieces completely.

Nutrition:

- Calories: 483
- Fats: 12.5 g
- Saturated Fats: 3.4 g
- Carbs: 35.1 g
- Fiber: 1.6 g
- Sugar: 1.8 g
- Protein: 53.7 g

Lemony Chicken Thighs

Preparation Time: 15 minutes
Cooking Time: 20 minutes
Servings: 6
Ingredients:

- 6 (6-oz.) chicken thighs
- 2 tbsp. olive oil
- 2 tbsp. fresh lemon juice

- 1 tbsp. Italian seasoning
- Salt and ground black pepper, as required
- 1 lemon, sliced thinly

Directions:

1. In a large bowl, add all the ingredients except for the lemon slices and toss to coat well.
2. Refrigerate to marinate for 30 minutes or overnight.
3. Remove the chicken thighs and let any excess marinade drip off.
4. Press the "Power" button of the Ninja Foodi Digital Air Fry Oven and turn the dial to select "Air Fry" mode.
5. Press the "Time" button and again turn the dial to set the cooking time to 20 minutes.
6. Now push the "Temp" button and rotate the dial to set the temperature at 350°F.
7. Press the "Start/Pause" button to start.
8. When the unit beeps to show that it is preheated, open the lid and grease the air fry basket.
9. Place the chicken thighs into the prepared air fry basket and insert them in the Air Fry Oven.
10. After 10 minutes of cooking, flip the chicken thighs.
11. When cooking time is completed, open the lid and serve hot alongside the lemon slices.

Serving Suggestions: Serve alongside your favorite dipping sauce.

Variation Tip: Select chicken with a pinkish hue.

Nutrition:

- Calories: 472
- Fats: 18 g
- Saturated Fats: 4.3 g
- Carbs: 0.6 g
- Fiber: 0.1 g
- Sugar: 0.4 g
- Protein: 49.3 g

Chinese Chicken Drumsticks

Preparation Time: 10 minutes
Cooking Time: 20 minutes
Servings: 4
Ingredients:

- 1 tbsp. oyster sauce
- 1 tsp. light soy sauce
- ½ tsp. sesame oil
- 1 tsp. Chinese five-spice powder

- Salt and ground black pepper, as required
- 4 (6-oz.) chicken drumsticks
- 1 cup corn flour

Directions:

1. In a bowl, mix together the sauces, oil, five-spice powder, salt, and black pepper.
2. Add the chicken drumsticks and coat them generously with the marinade.
3. Refrigerate for at least 30–40 minutes.
4. In a shallow dish, place the corn flour.
5. Remove the chicken from marinade and lightly coat with corn flour.
6. Press the "Power" button of the Ninja Foodi Digital Air Fry Oven and turn the dial to select "Air Fry" mode.
7. Press the "Time" button and again turn the dial to set the cooking time to 20 minutes.
8. Now push the "Temp" button and rotate the dial to set the temperature at 390°F.
9. Press the "Start/Pause" button to start.
10. When the unit beeps to show that it is preheated, open the lid and grease the air fry basket.
11. Place the chicken drumsticks into the prepared air fry basket and insert them in the Air Fry Oven.
12. When the cooking time is completed, open the lid and serve hot.

Serving Suggestions: Serve with fresh greens.

Variation Tip: Use best quality sauces.

Nutrition:

- Calories: 287
- Fats: 13.8 g
- Saturated Fats: 7.1 g
- Carbs: 1.6 g
- Fiber: 0.2 g
- Sugar: 0.1 g
- Protein: 38.3 g

Crispy Chicken Thighs

Preparation Time: 15 minutes
Cooking Time: 25 minutes
Servings: 4
Ingredients:

- ½ cup all-purpose flour
- 1½ tbsp. Cajun seasoning
- 1 tsp. seasoning salt
- 1 egg

- 4 (4-oz.) chicken thighs, skin-on

Directions:

1. In a shallow bowl, mix together the flour, Cajun seasoning, and seasoning salt.
2. In another bowl, crack the egg and beat well.
3. Coat each chicken thigh with the flour mixture, then dip them into the beaten egg and finally, coat them with the flour mixture again.
4. Shake off the excess flour thoroughly.
5. Press the "Power" button of the Ninja Foodi Digital Air Fry Oven and turn the dial to select "Air Fry" mode.
6. Press the "Time" and again turn the dial to set the cooking time to 25 minutes.
7. Now push the "Temp" and rotate the dial to set the temperature at 390°F.
8. Press the "Start/Pause" button to start.
9. When the unit beeps to show that it is preheated, open the lid and grease the air fry basket.
10. Place the chicken thighs into the prepared air fry basket and insert them in the Air Fry Oven.
11. When cooking time is completed, open the lid and serve hot.

Serving Suggestions: Serve with ketchup.

Variation Tip: Feel free to use seasoning of your choice.

Nutrition:
- Calories: 288
- Fats: 9.6 g
- Saturated Fats: 2.7 g
- Carbs: 12 g
- Fiber: 0.4 g
- Sugar: 0.1 g
- Protein: 35.9 g

Oat Crusted Chicken Breasts

Preparation Time: 15 minutes

Cooking Time: 12 minutes

Servings: 2

Ingredients:
- 2 (6-oz.) chicken breasts
- Salt and ground black pepper, as required
- ¾ cup oats
- 2 tbsp. mustard powder
- 1 tbsp. fresh parsley
- 2 medium eggs

Directions:

1. Place the chicken breasts onto a cutting board, and with a meat mallet, flatten each into an even thickness.
2. Then, cut each chicken breast in half.
3. Sprinkle the chicken pieces with salt and black pepper and set aside.
4. In a blender, add the oats, mustard powder, parsley, salt and black pepper and pulse until a coarse breadcrumb-like mixture is formed.
5. Transfer the oat mixture into a shallow bowl.
6. In another bowl, crack the eggs and beat well.
7. Coat the chicken with oat mixture, dip into beaten eggs, and coat with the oat mixture again.
8. Press the "Power" button of the Ninja Foodi Digital Air Fry Oven and turn the dial to select "Air Fry" mode.
9. Press the "Time" button and again turn the dial to set the cooking time to 12 minutes.
10. Now push the "Temp" and rotate the dial to set the temperature at 350°F.
11. Press the "Start/Pause" button to start.
12. When the unit beeps to show that it is preheated, open the lid and grease the air fry basket.
13. Place the chicken breasts into the prepared air fry basket and insert them in the Air Fry Oven.
14. Flip the chicken breasts once halfway through.
15. When cooking time is completed, open the lid and serve hot.

Serving Suggestions: Serve with mashed potatoes.

Variation Tip: Check the meat "best by" date.

Nutrition:
- Calories: 556
- Fats: 22.2 g
- Saturated Fats: 5.3 g
- Carbs: 25.1 g
- Fiber: 4.8 g
- Sugar: 1.4 g
- Protein: 61.6 g

Crispy Chicken Cutlets

Preparation Time: 15 minutes

Cooking Time: 30 minutes

Servings: 4

Ingredients:

- ¾ cup flour
- 2 large eggs
- 1½ cups breadcrumbs
- ¼ cup Parmesan cheese, grated
- 1 tbsp. mustard powder
- Salt and ground black pepper, as required
- 4 (6-oz.) (¼-inch thick) skinless, boneless chicken cutlets

Directions:

1. In a shallow bowl, add the flour.
2. In a second bowl, crack the eggs and beat them well.
3. In a third bowl, mix together the breadcrumbs, cheese, mustard powder, salt, and black pepper.
4. Season the chicken with salt, and black pepper.
5. Coat the chicken with flour, then dip them into beaten eggs and finally coat them with the breadcrumbs mixture.
6. Press the "Power" button of the Ninja Foodi Digital Air Fry Oven and turn the dial to select "Air Fry" mode.
7. Press the "Time" button and again turn the dial to set the cooking time to 30 minutes.
8. Now push the "Temp" button and rotate the dial to set the temperature at 355°F.
9. Press the "Start/Pause" button to start.
10. When the unit beeps to show that it is preheated, open the lid and grease the air fry basket.
11. Place the chicken cutlets into the prepared air fry basket and insert them in the Air Fry Oven.
12. When the cooking time is completed, open the lid and serve hot.

Serving Suggestions: Serve with favorite greens.
Variation Tip: Parmesan cheese can be replaced with your favorite cheese.

Nutrition:

- Calories: 526
- Fats: 13 g
- Saturated Fats: 4.2 g
- Carbs: 48.6 g
- Fiber: 3 g
- Sugar: 3 g
- Protein: 51.7 g

Brie Stuffed Chicken Breasts

Preparation Time: 15 minutes
Cooking Time: 15 minutes
Servings: 4
Ingredients:

- 2 (8-oz.) skinless, boneless chicken fillets
- Salt and ground black pepper, as required
- 4 brie cheese slices
- 1 tbsp. fresh chive, minced
- 4 bacon slices

Directions:

1. Cut each chicken fillet in 2 equal-sized pieces.
2. Carefully, make a slit in each chicken piece horizontally, about ¼-inch from the edge.
3. Open each chicken piece and season them with salt and black pepper.
4. Place 1 cheese slice in the open area of each chicken piece and sprinkle with the chives.
5. Close the chicken pieces and wrap each one with a bacon slice.
6. Secure with toothpicks.
7. Press the "Power" button of th Ninja Foodi Digital Air Fry Oven and turn the dial to select "Air Fry" mode.
8. Press the "Time" button and again turn the dial to set the cooking time to 15 minutes.
9. Now push the "Temp" button and rotate the dial to set the temperature at 355°F.
10. Press the "Start/Pause" button to start.
11. When the unit beeps to show that it is preheated, open the lid and grease the air fry basket.
12. Place the chicken pieces into the prepared air fry basket and insert them in the oven.
13. When the cooking time is completed, open the lid and place the rolled chicken breasts onto a cutting board.
14. Cut into desired slice sizes and serve.

Serving Suggestions: Serve with creamy mashed potatoes.
Variation Tip: Season the chicken breasts slightly.
Nutrition:

- Calories: 394
- Fats: 24 g
- Saturated Fats: 10.4 g
- Carbs: 0.6 g
- Sugar: 0.1 g
- Protein: 42 g

Chicken Kabobs

Preparation Time: 15 minutes
Cooking Time: 9 minutes
Servings: 2
Ingredients:

- 1 (8-oz.) chicken breast, cut into medium-sized pieces
- 1 tbsp. fresh lemon juice
- 3 garlic cloves, grated
- 1 tbsp. fresh oregano, minced
- ½ tsp. lemon zest, grated
- Salt and ground black pepper, as required
- 1 tsp. plain Greek yogurt
- 1 tsp. olive oil

Directions:

1. In a large bowl, add the chicken, lemon juice, garlic, oregano, lemon zest, salt and black pepper and toss to coat well.
2. Cover the bowl and refrigerate overnight.
3. Remove the bowl from the refrigerator and stir in the yogurt and oil.
4. Thread the chicken pieces onto the metal skewers.
5. Press the "Power" button of the Ninja Foodi Digital Air Fry Oven and turn the dial to select "Air Fry" mode.
6. Press the "Time" button and again turn the dial to set the cooking time to 9 minutes.
7. Now push the "Temp" button and rotate the dial to set the temperature at 350°F.
8. Press "Start/Pause" button to start.
9. When the unit beeps to show that it is preheated, open the lid and grease the air fry basket.
10. Place the skewers into the prepared air fry basket and insert them in the oven.
11. Flip the skewers once halfway through.
12. When cooking time is completed, open the lid and serve hot.

Serving Suggestions: Serve alongside fresh salad.
Variation Tip: Make sure to tri the chicken pieces.
Nutrition:

- Calories: 167
- Fats: 5.5 g
- Saturated Fats: 0.5 g
- Carbs: 3.4 g
- Fiber: 0.5 g
- Sugar: 1.1 g
- Protein: 24.8 g

Simple Turkey Breast

Preparation Time: 10 minutes
Cooking Time: 1 hour 20 minutes
Servings: 6
Ingredients:

- 1 (2 ¾-lb.) turkey breast half, bone-in, skin-on
- Salt and ground black pepper, as required

Directions:

1. Rub the turkey breast with the salt and black pepper evenly.
2. Arrange the turkey breast into a greased baking pan.
3. Press the "Power" button of the Ninja Foodi Digital Air Fry Oven and turn the dial to select "Air Bake" mode.
4. Press the "Time" and again turn the dial to set the cooking time to 1 hour 20 minutes.
5. Now push the "Temp" button and rotate the dial to set the temperature at 450ºF.
6. Press the "Start/Pause" button to start.
7. Open the unit when it has reached the temperature, when it beeps.
8. Arrange the pan over the wire rack and insert it in the oven.
9. When cooking time is completed, open the lid and place the turkey breast onto a cutting board.
10. With a piece of foil, cover the turkey breast for about 20 minutes before slicing.
11. With a sharp knife, cut the turkey breast into desired size slices and serve.

Serving Suggestions: Serve alongside the steamed veggies.
Variation Tip: Beware of flat spots on meat, which can indicate thawing and refreezing.
Nutrition:

- Calories: 221
- Fats: 0.8 g
- Protein: 51.6 g

Herbed Duck Breast

Preparation Time: 15 minutes
Cooking Time: 20 minutes
Servings: 2

Ingredients:

- 1 (10-oz.) duck breast
- Olive oil cooking spray
- ½ tbsp. fresh thyme, chopped
- ½ tbsp. fresh rosemary, chopped
- 1 cup chicken broth
- 1 tbsp. fresh lemon juice
- Salt and ground black pepper, as required

Directions:

1. Spray the duck breast with cooking spray evenly.
2. In a bowl, mix well the remaining ingredients.
3. Add the duck breast and coat it with the marinade generously.
4. Refrigerate it covered for about 4 hours.
5. With a piece of foil, cover the duck breast.
6. Press the "Power" of the Ninja Foodi Digital Air Fry Oven and turn the dial to select "Air Fry" mode.
7. Press the "Time" button and again turn the dial to set the cooking time to 15 minutes.
8. Now push the "Temp" and rotate the dial to set the temperature at 390ºF.
9. Press the "Start/Pause" button to start.
10. When the unit beeps to show that it is preheated, open the lid and grease the air fry basket.
11. Place the duck breast into the prepared air fry basket and insert them in the Air Fry Oven.
12. After 15 minutes of cooking, set the temperature to 355ºF for 5 minutes.
13. When the cooking time is completed, open the lid and serve hot.

Serving Suggestions: Serve with spiced potatoes.

Variation Tip: Don't undercook the duck meat.

Nutrition:

- Calories: 209
- Fats: 6.6 g
- Saturated Fats: 0.3 g
- Carbs: 1.6 g
- Fiber: 0.6 g
- Sugar: 0.5 g
- Protein: 33.8 g

CHAPTER 6: VEGETABLES AND SIDES

Crispy Brussels Sprouts

Preparation Time: 5 minutes
Cooking Time: 10 minutes
Servings: 2
Ingredients:

- ½ lb.Brussels sprouts, cut in half
- ½ tbsp. oil
- ½ tbsp. unsalted butter, melted

Directions:

1. Rub the sprouts with oil.
2. Place them into the air fry basket.
3. Cook at 400ºF for 10 minutes. Stir once at the halfway mark.
4. Remove the air fry basket and drizzle with the melted butter.
5. Serve.

Nutrition:

- Calories: 90
- Fats: 6.1 g
- Carb: 4 g
- Protein: 2.9 g

Flatbread

Preparation Time: 5 minutes
Cooking Time: 7 minutes
Servings: 2
Ingredients:

- 1 cup shredded mozzarella cheese
- ¼ cup almond flour
- 1 oz. full-fat cream cheese, softened

Directions:

1. Melt the mozzarella in the microwave for 30 seconds. Stir in the almond flour until smooth.
2. Add the cream cheese. Continue mixing until a dough forms. Knead with your wet hands if necessary.
3. Divide the dough into two pieces and roll out to ¼-inch thickness between two pieces of parchment.
4. Cover the air fry basket with parchment and place the flatbreads into the air fry basket. Work in batches if necessary.
5. Cook at 320ºF for 7 minutes. Flip once at the halfway mark.
6. Serve.

Nutrition:

- Calories: 296
- Fats: 22.6 g
- Carb: 3.3 g
- Protein: 16.3 g

Creamy Cabbage

Preparation Time: 10 minutes
Cooking Time: 20 minutes
Servings: 2
Ingredients:

- ½ green cabbage head, chopped
- ½ yellow onion, chopped
- Salt and black pepper, to taste
- ½ cup whipped cream
- 1 tbsp. cornstarch

Directions:

1. Put the cabbage and the onion in the Air Fry Oven.
2. In a bowl, mix cornstarch with the whipped cream, salt, and pepper. Stir and pour over cabbage.
3. Toss and cook at 400ºF for 20 minutes.
4. Serve.

Nutrition:

- Calories: 208
- Fats: 10 g
- Carb: 16 g
- Protein: 5 g

Creamy Potatoes

Preparation Time: 10 minutes
Cooking Time: 20 minutes
Servings: 2
Ingredients:

- ¾ lb. potatoes, peeled and cubed
- 1 tbsp. olive oil
- Salt and black pepper, to taste
- ½ tbsp. hot paprika
- ½ cup Greek yogurt
- 1 cup Water

Directions:

1. Place the potatoes in a bowl, pour the water to cover, and leave aside for 10 minutes. Drain, pat dry and transfer to another bowl.

2. Add the salt, pepper, paprika, and half of the oil to the potatoes and mix.

3. Put the potatoes in the air fry basket and cook at 360ºF for 20 minutes.

4. In a bowl, mix the yogurt with salt, pepper, and the rest of the oil and whisk.

5. Divide the potatoes onto plates, drizzle with yogurt dressing, mix, and serve.

Nutrition:
- Calories: 170
- Fats: 3 g
- Carb: 20 g
- Protein: 5 g

Green Beans and Cherry Tomatoes

Preparation Time: 10 minutes
Cooking Time: 15 minutes
Servings: 2
Ingredients:
- 8 oz. cherry tomatoes
- 8 oz. green beans
- 1 tbsp. olive oil
- Salt and black pepper, to taste

Directions:
1. In a bowl, mix the cherry tomatoes with green beans, olive oil, salt, and pepper. Mix.

2. Cook in the air fryer at 400ºF for 15 minutes. Shake once.

3. Serve.

Nutrition:
- Calories: 162
- Fats: 6 g
- Carb: 8 g
- Protein: 9 g

Crispy Brussels Sprouts and Potatoes

Preparation Time: 10 minutes
Cooking Time: 8 minutes
Servings: 2
Ingredients:
- ¾ lb. Brussels sprouts, washed and trimmed
- ½ cup new potatoes, chopped
- 2 tsp. breadcrumbs
- Salt and black pepper, to taste
- 2 tsp. butter

Directions:

1. In a bowl, add the Brussels sprouts, potatoes, bread crumbs, salt, pepper, and butter. Mix well.

2. Place the mixture in the Air Fry Oven and cook at 400ºF for 8 minutes.

3. Serve.

Nutrition:
- Calories: 152
- Fats: 3 g
- Carb: 17 g
- Protein: 4 g

Herbed Tomatoes

Preparation Time: 10 minutes
Cooking Time: 15 minutes
Servings: 2
Ingredients:
- 2 big tomatoes, halved and insides scooped out
- Salt and black pepper, to taste
- ½ tbsp. olive oil
- 1 garlic clove, minced
- ¼ tsp. thyme, chopped

Directions:
1. In the air fry basket, mix the tomatoes with thyme, garlic, oil, salt, and pepper.

2. Mix and cook at 390ºF for 15 minutes.

3. Serve.

Nutrition:
- Calories: 112
- Fats: 1 g
- Carb: 4 g
- Protein: 4 g

Air Fried Leeks

Preparation Time: 10 minutes
Cooking Time: 7 minutes
Servings: 2
Ingredients:
- 2 leeks, washed, ends cut, and halved
- Salt and black pepper, to taste
- ½ tbsp. butter, melted
- ½ tbsp. lemon juice

Directions:
1. Rub the leeks with the melted butter and season with salt and pepper.

2.   Lay them inside the air fryer and cook at 350ºF for 7 minutes.

3.   Arrange them on a platter. Drizzle them with the lemon juice and serve.

Nutrition:
- Calories: 100
- Fats: 4 g
- Carb: 6 g
- Protein: 2 g

Crispy Broccoli

Preparation Time: 10 minutes
Cooking Time: 10 minutes
Servings: 4
Ingredients:
- 1 large head fresh broccoli
- 2 tsp. olive oil
- 2 tpsp Lemon juice

Directions:
1.   Rinse the broccoli and pat it dry. Cut off the florets and separate them (you can also use the broccoli stems too). Cut them into 1-inch chunks and peel them.

2.   Toss the broccoli, olive oil, and lemon juice in a large bowl until coated.

3.   Roast the broccoli in the Air Fry Basket in batches for 10–14 minutes or until the broccoli is crisp-tender and slightly brown around the edges. Repeat with the remaining broccoli. Serve immediately.

Nutrition:
- Calories: 63
- Fats: 2 g
- Protein: 4 g
- Carbs: 10 g
- Sodium: 50 mg
- Fiber: 4 g

Garlic-Roasted Bell Peppers

Preparation Time: 5 minutes
Cooking Time: 20 minutes
Servings: 4
Ingredients:
- 4 bell peppers, any colors, stemmed, seeded, membranes removed, and cut into fourths
- 1 tsp. olive oil
- 4 garlic cloves, minced
- ½ tsp. dried thyme

Directions:
1.   Put the peppers in the air fry basket and drizzle with olive oil. Toss gently. Roast for 15 minutes.

2.   Sprinkle with the garlic and thyme. Roast for 3–5 minutes more, or until tender. Serve immediately.

Nutrition:
- Calories: 36
- Fats: 1 g
- Protein: 1 g
- Carbs: 5 g
- Sodium: 21 mg
- Fiber: 2 g

Asparagus with Garlic

Preparation Time: 5 minutes
Cooking Time: 10 minutes
Servings: 4
Ingredients:
- 1-lb. asparagus, rinsed, ends snapped off where they naturally break (see Tip)
- 2 tsp. olive oil
- 3 garlic cloves, minced
- 2 tbsp. balsamic vinegar
- ½ tsp. dried thyme

Directions:
1.   In a huge bowl, mix the asparagus with olive oil. -Transfer to the air fry basket.

2.   Sprinkle with garlic. Roast for 4–5 minutes for crisp-tender or for 8–11 minutes for the asparagus to get crisp on the outside and tender on the inside.

3.   Drizzle with the balsamic vinegar and the thyme leaves. Serve immediately.

Nutrition:
- Calories: 41
- Fats: 1 g
- Protein: 3 g
- Carbs: 6 g
- Sodium: 3 mg

Cheesy Roasted Sweet Potatoes

Preparation Time: 5 minutes
Cooking Time: 20 minutes
Servings: 4

Ingredients:
- 2 large sweet potatoes, peeled and sliced
- 1 tsp. olive oil
- 1 tbsp. white balsamic vinegar
- 1 tsp. dried thyme
- ¼ cup grated Parmesan cheese

Directions:
1. In a big bowl, shower the sweet potato slices with the olive oil and toss.
2. Sprinkle with the balsamic vinegar and thyme and toss again.
3. Sprinkle the potatoes with the Parmesan cheese and toss to coat.
4. Roast the slices in the air fryer basket in batches for 18–23 minutes, tossing the sweet potato slices in the basket during cooking, until tender.
5. Repeat with the remaining sweet potato slices. Serve immediately.

Nutrition:
- Calories: 100
- Fats: 3 g
- Protein: 4 g
- Carbs: 15 g
- Sodium: 132 mg

Salty Lemon Artichokes

Preparation Time: 15 minutes
Cooking Time: 45 minutes
Servings: 2
Ingredients:
- 1 lemon
- 2 artichokes
- 1 tsp. kosher salt
- 1 garlic head
- 2 tsp. olive oil

Directions:
1. Cut off the edges of the artichokes.
2. Cut the lemon into the halves.
3. Peel the garlic head and chop the garlic cloves roughly.
4. Then place the chopped garlic in the artichokes.
5. Sprinkle the artichokes with the olive oil and kosher salt.
6. Then squeeze the lemon juice into the artichokes.
7. Wrap the artichokes in the foil.
8. Preheat the Air Fry Oven to 330ºF.
9. Place the wrapped artichokes in the air fryer and cook for 45 minutes.
10. When the artichokes are cooked, discard the foil and serve.
11. Enjoy!

Nutrition:
- Calories: 133
- Fats: 5 g
- Fiber: 9.7 g
- Carbs: 21.7 g
- Protein: 6 g

Asparagus & Parmesan

Preparation Time: 10 minutes
Cooking Time: 6 minutes
Servings: 2
Ingredients:
- 1 tsp. sesame oil
- 11 oz. asparagus
- 1 tsp. chicken stock
- ½ tsp. ground white pepper
- 3 oz. Parmesan

Directions:
1. Wash the asparagus and chop them roughly.
2. Sprinkle the chopped asparagus with the chicken stock and ground white pepper.
3. Then sprinkle the asparagus with the sesame oil and shake them.
4. Place the asparagus in the air fry basket.
5. Cook the vegetables for 4 minutes at 400ºF.
6. Meanwhile, shred the Parmesan cheese.
7. When the time is over, shake the asparagus gently and sprinkle with the shredded cheese.
8. Cook the asparagus for 2 minutes more at 400ºF.
9. After this, transfer the cooked asparagus in the serving plates.
10. Serve and taste it!

Nutrition:
- Calories: 189
- Fats: 11.6 g
- Fiber: 3.4 g
- Carbs: 7.9 g
- Protein: 17.2 g

Corn on Cobs

Preparation Time: 10 minutes
Cooking Time: 10 minutes
Servings: 2
Ingredients:
- 2 fresh corn on cobs
- 2 tsp. butter
- 1 tsp. salt
- 1 tsp. paprika
- ¼ tsp. olive oil

Directions:
1. Preheat the Air Fry Oven to 400ºF.
2. Rub the corn on cobs with the salt and paprika.
3. Then sprinkle the corn on cobs with the olive oil.
4. Place the corn on cobs in the air fry basket.
5. Cook the corn on cobs for 10 minutes.
6. When the time is over, transfer the corn on cobs in the serving plates and rub with the butter gently.
7. Serve the meal immediately.
8. Enjoy!

Nutrition:
- Calories: 122
- Fats: 5.5 g
- Fiber: 2.4 g
- Carbs: 17.6 g
- Protein: 3.2 g

Onion Green Beans

Preparation Time: 10 minutes
Cooking Time: 12 minutes
Servings: 2
Ingredients:
- 11 oz green beans
- 1 tbsp. onion powder
- 1 tbsp. olive oil
- ½ tsp. salt
- ¼ tsp. chili flakes

Directions:
1. Wash the green beans carefully and place them in a bowl.
2. Sprinkle the green beans with the onion powder, salt, chili flakes, and olive oil.
3. Shake the green beans carefully.
4. Preheat the Air Fry Oven to 400ºF.
5. Put the green beans in the Air Fry Oven and cook for 8 minutes.
6. After this, shake the green beans and cook them for 4 minutes more at 400ºF.
7. When the time is over, shake the green beans.
8. Serve the side dish and enjoy!

Nutrition:
- Calories: 1205
- Fats: 7.2 g
- Fiber: 5.5 g
- Carbs: 13.9 g
- Protein: 3.2 g

Dill Mashed Potato

Preparation Time: 10 minutes
Cooking Time: 15 minutes
Servings: 2
Ingredients:
- 2 potatoes
- 2 tbsp. fresh dill, chopped
- 1 tsp. butter
- ½ tsp. salt
- ¼ cup half and half

Directions:
1. Preheat the air fryer to 390ºF.
2. Rinse the potatoes thoroughly and place them in the Air Fry Oven.
3. Cook the potatoes for 15 minutes.
4. After this, remove the potatoes from the Air Fry Oven.
5. Peel the potatoes.
6. Mash the potatoes well with the help of the fork.
7. Then add the chopped fresh dill and salt.
8. Stir it gently and add the butter and half and half.
9. Take the hand blender and blend the mixture well.
10. When the mashed potato is cooked, serve it immediately. Enjoy!

Nutrition:
- Calories: 211
- Fats: 5.7 g
- Fiber: 5.5 g
- Carbs: 36.5 g
- Protein: 5.1 g

Cream Potato

Preparation Time: 15 minutes
Cooking Time: 20 minutes
Servings: 2
Ingredients:

- 3 medium potatoes, scrubbed
- ½ tsp. kosher salt
- 1 tbsp. Italian seasoning
- ⅓ cup cream
- ½ tsp. ground black pepper

Directions:

1. Slice the potatoes.
2. Preheat the air fryer to 365 F.
3. Make the first layer from the sliced potato in the air fry basket.
4. Sprinkle the potato layer with the kosher salt and ground black pepper.
5. After this, make the second layer of the potato and sprinkle it with the Italian seasoning.
6. Make the last layer of the sliced potato and pour the cream.
7. Cook the scallop potato for 20 minutes.
8. When the scalloped potato is cooked, let it chill till the room temperature. Enjoy!

Nutrition:

- Calories: 269
- Fats: 4.7 g
- Fiber: 7.8 g
- Carbs: 52.6 g
- Protein: 5.8 g

Chili Squash Wedges

Preparation Time: 10 minutes
Cooking Time: 18 minutes
Servings: 2
Ingredients:

- 11 oz Acorn squash
- ½ tsp. salt
- 1 tbsp. olive oil
- ½ tsp. chili pepper
- ½ tsp. paprika

Directions:

1. Cut the Acorn squash into the wedges.
2. Sprinkle the wedges with the salt, olive oil, chili pepper, and paprika.
3. Massage the wedges gently.
4. Preheat the Air Fry Oven to 400ºF.
5. Put the Acorn squash wedges in the air fry basket and cook for 18 minutes.
6. Flip the wedges onto another side after 9 minutes of cooking.
7. Serve the cooked meal hot. Enjoy!

Nutrition:

- Calories: 125
- Fats: 7.2 g
- Fiber: 2.6 g
- Carbs: 16.7 g
- Protein: 1.4 g

Honey Carrots with Greens

Preparation Time: 7 minutes
Cooking Time: 12 minutes
Servings: 2
Ingredients:

- 1 cup baby carrot
- ½ tsp. salt
- ½ tsp. white pepper
- 1 tbsp. honey
- 1 tsp. sesame oil

Directions:

1. Preheat the Air Fry Oven to 385ºF.
2. Combine the baby carrot with the salt, white pepper, and sesame oil.
3. Shake the baby carrot and transfer in the air fry basket.
4. Cook the vegetables for 10 minutes.
5. After this, add the honey and shake the carrots.
6. Cook the meal for 2 minutes.
7. After this, shake the carrots and serve immediately.
8. Enjoy!

Nutrition:

- Calories: 83
- Fats: 2.4 g
- Fiber: 2.6 g
- Carbs: 16 g
- Protein: 0.6 g

South Asian Cauliflower Fritters

Preparation Time: 5 minutes
Cooking Time: 20 minutes
Servings: 4
Ingredients:

- 1 large chopped into florets cauliflower
- 3 tbsp. Greek yogurt
- 3 tbsp. flour
- ½ tsp. ground turmeric
- ½ tsp. ground cumin
- ½ tsp. ground paprika
- 12 tsp. ground coriander
- ½ tsp. salt
- ½ tsp. black pepper

Directions:

1. Using a large bowl, add and mix the Greek yogurt, flour, and seasonings properly.
2. Add the cauliflower florets and toss it until it is well covered
3. Heat up your air fryer to 390ºF.
4. Grease your air fry basket with a non-stick cooking spray and add half of the cauliflower florets to it.
5. Cook it for 10 minutes or until it turns golden brown and crispy, then shake it after 5 minutes. (Repeat this with the other half).
6. Serve and enjoy!

Nutrition:
- Calories: 120
- Fats: 4 g
- Protein: 7.5 g
- Carbs: 14 g
- Fiber: 3.4 g

Supreme Air-Fried Tofu

Preparation Time: 5 minutes
Cooking Time: 50 minutes
Servings: 4
Ingredients:
- 1 block extra-firm tofu, pressed and sliced into 1-inch cubes
- 2 tbsp. soy sauce
- 1 tsp. seasoned rice vinegar
- 2 tsp. toasted sesame oil
- 1 tbsp. cornstarch

Directions:

1. Using a bowl, add and toss the tofu, soy sauce, seasoned rice vinegar, sesame oil until they are properly covered.
2. Place it inside your refrigerator and allow to marinate for 30 minutes.
3. Preheat your air fryer to 370ºF.
4. Add the cornstarch to the tofu mixture and toss it until it is properly covered.
5. Grease your air fryer basket with a non-stick cooking spray and add the tofu inside the basket.
6. Cook it for 20 minutes at a 370ºF, and shake it after 10 minutes.
7. Serve and enjoy!

Nutrition:
- Calories: 80
- Fats: 5.8 g
- Protein: 5 g
- Carbs: 3 g
- Fiber: 1.2 g

Not Your Average Zucchini Parmesan Chips

Preparation Time: 5 minutes
Cooking Time: 10 minutes
Servings: 4
Ingredients:
- 2 thinly sliced zucchinis
- 1 beaten egg
- ½ cup panko breadcrumbs
- ½ cup grated Parmesan cheese
- Salt and black pepper

Directions:

1. Prepare the zucchini by using a mandolin or a knife to slice them thinly.
2. Use a cloth to pat dry the zucchini chips.
3. Then using a bowl, add the egg and beat it properly. After that, pick another bowl, and add the breadcrumbs, Parmesan cheese, salt, and black pepper.
4. Dredge the zucchini chips into the egg mixture and then cover it with the Parmesan-breadcrumb mixture.
5. Grease the battered zucchini chips with a non-stick cooking spray and place it inside your Air Fry Oven.
6. Cook it for 8 minutes at 350ºF.
7. Once done, carefully remove it from your Air Fry Oven and sprinkle another tsp. of salt to give it some taste. Serve and enjoy!

Nutrition:
- Calories: 100
- Fats: 6 g

- Protein: 4 g
- Carbs: 9 g
- Fiber: 1.8 g

Sky-High Roasted Corn

Preparation Time: 5 minutes
Cooking Time: 10 minutes
Servings: 4
Ingredients:

- 4 ears of husk-less corn
- 1 tbsp. olive oil
- 1 tsp. salt
- 1 tsp. black pepper

Directions:

1. Heat up your Air Fry Oven to 400ºF.
2. Sprinkle the ears of corn with the olive oil, salt and black pepper.
3. Place it inside your air fryer and cook it for 10 minutes at 400ºF.
4. Serve and enjoy!

Nutrition:

- Calories: 100
- Fats: 1 g
- Protein: 3 g
- Fiber: 3 g
- Carbs: 22 g

Ravishing Air-Fried Carrots with Honey Glaze

Preparation Time: 5 minutes
Cooking Time: 10 minutes
Servings: 1
Ingredients:

- 3 cups carrots chopped into ½-inch pieces
- 1 tbsp. olive oil
- 2 tbsp. honey
- 1 tbsp. brown sugar
- Salt and black pepper

Directions:

1. Heat up your Air Fry Oven to 390ºF.
2. Using a bowl, add and toss the carrot pieces, olive oil, honey, brown sugar, salt, and the black pepper until the carrots are properly covered.
3. Place it inside your Air Fry Oven and add the carrots.
4. Cook it for 12 minutes at 390ºF, and then shake after 6 minutes. Serve and enjoy!

Nutrition:

- Calories: 90
- Fats: 3.5 g
- Fiber: 2 g
- Carbs: 13 g
- Protein: 1 g

Flaming Buffalo Cauliflower Bites

Preparation Time: 5 minutes
Cooking Time: 20 minutes
Servings: 4
Ingredients:

- 1 cauliflower head, large and chopped into florets
- 3 beaten eggs
- 2/3 cup cornstarch
- 2 tbsp. melted butter
- ¼ cup hot sauce

Directions:

1. Heat up your Air Fry Oven to 360ºF.
2. Using a large mixing bowl, add and mix the eggs and the cornstarch a properly.
3. Add the cauliflower, gently toss it until it is properly covered with the batter, shake it off in case of any excess batter and set it aside.
4. Grease your air fry basket with a non-stick cooking spray and add the cauliflower bites, which will require you to work in batches.
5. Cook the cauliflower bites for 15–20 minutes or until it has a golden-brown color and a crispy texture, while still shaking occasionally.
6. Then, in a small mixing bowl, add and mix the melted butter and hot sauce properly.
7. Once the cauliflower bites are done, remove it from your Air Fry Oven and place it into a large bowl. Pour the buffalo sauce over the cauliflower bites and toss it until it is properly covered.
8. Serve and enjoy!

Nutrition:

- Calories: 240
- Fats: 5.5 g
- Fiber: 6.3 g
- Protein: 8.8 g
- Carbs: 37 g

Pleasant Air-Fried Eggplant

Preparation Time: 5 minutes

Cooking Time: 20 minutes
Servings: 4
Ingredients:

- 2 eggplants, thinly sliced or chopped into chunks
- 1 tsp. salt
- 1 tsp. black pepper
- 1 cup rice flour
- 1 cup white wine

Directions:

1. In a bowl, add the rice flour, white wine and mix properly until it gets smooth.
2. Add the salt, black pepper and stir again.
3. Dredge the eggplant slices or chunks into the batter and remove any excess batter.
4. Heat up your Air Fry Oven to 390ºF.
5. Grease the air fry basket with a non-stick cooking spray.
6. Add the eggplant slices or chunks into your Air Fry Oven and cook it for 15–20 minutes or until it has a golden brown and crispy texture, while still shaking it occasionally.
7. Carefully, remove it from your air fryer and allow it to cool off. Serve and enjoy!

Nutrition:

- Calories: 380
- Fats: 15 g
- Protein: 13 g
- Fiber: 6.1 g
- Carbs: 51 g

Cauliflower Hash

Preparation Time: 10 minutes
Cooking Time: 15 minutes
Servings: 6
Ingredients:

- 1 lb. cauliflower
- 2 eggs
- 1 tsp. salt
- ½ tsp. ground paprika
- 4 oz. turkey fillet, chopped

Directions:

1. Wash the cauliflower, chop, and set aside.
2. In a different bowl, crack the eggs and whisk well.
3. Add the salt and ground paprika and stir.

4. Place the chopped turkey in the air fryer basket and cook it for 4 minutes at 365° F, stirring halfway through.
5. After this, add the chopped cauliflower and stir the mixture.
6. Cook the turkey-cauliflower mixture for 6 minutes more at 370°F, stirring it halfway through.
7. Then pour in the whisked egg mixture and stir it carefully.
8. Cook the cauliflower hash for 5 minutes more at 365°F.
9. When the cauliflower hash is done, let it cool and transfer to serving bowls. Serve and enjoy!

Nutrition:

- Calories: 143 g
- Fats: 9.5 g
- Fiber: 2 g
- Carbs: 4.5 g
- Protein: 10.4 g

Asparagus with Almonds

Preparation Time: 10 minutes
Cooking Time: 5 minutes
Servings: 2
Ingredients:

- 9 oz. asparagus
- 1 tsp. almond flour
- 1 tbsp. almond flakes
- ¼ tsp. salt
- 1 tsp. olive oil

Directions:

1. Combine the almond flour and almond flakes and stir the mixture well.
2. Sprinkle the asparagus with the olive oil and salt.
3. Shake it gently and coat in the almond flour mixture.
4. Place the asparagus in the air fry basket and cook at 400°F for 5 minutes, stirring halfway through.
5. Then cool a little and serve.

Nutrition:

- Calories: 143 g
- Fats: 11 g
- Fiber: 4.6 g
- Carbs: 8.6 g
- Protein: 6.4 g

Zucchini Cubes

Preparation Time: 7 minutes
Cooking Time: 8 minutes
Servings: 2
Ingredients:

- 1 zucchini
- ½ tsp. ground black pepper
- 1 tsp. oregano
- 2 tbsp. chicken stock
- ½ tsp. coconut oil

Directions:

1. Chop the zucchini into cubes.
2. Combine the ground black pepper, and oregano; stir the mixture.
3. Sprinkle the zucchini cubes with the spice mixture and stir well.
4. After this, sprinkle the zuchini with the chicken stock.
5. Place the coconut oil in the air fry basket and preheat it to 360°F for 20 seconds.
6. Then add the zucchini cubes and cook them for 8 minutes at 390°F, stirring halfway through.
7. Transfer to serving plates and enjoy!

Nutrition:

- Calories: 30
- Fats: 1.5 g
- Fiber: 1.6 g
- Carbs: 4.3 g
- Protein: 1.4 g

Sweet Potato & Onion Mix

Preparation Time: 10 minutes
Cooking Time: 15 minutes
Servings: 4
Ingredients:

- 2 sweet potatoes, peeled
- 1 red onion, peeled
- 1 white onion, peeled
- 1 tsp. olive oil
- ¼ cup almond milk

Directions:

1. Chop the sweet potatoes and the onions into cubes.
2. Sprinkle the sweet potatoes with olive oil.
3. Place the sweet potatoes in the air fry basket and cook for 5 minutes at 400°F.
4. Then stir the sweet potatoes and add the chopped onions.
5. Pour in the almond milk and stir gently.
6. Cook the mix for 10 minutes more at 400°F.
7. When the mix is cooked, let it cool a little and serve.

Nutrition:

- Calories: 56
- Fats: 4.8 g
- Fiber: 0.9 g
- Carbs: 3.5 g
- Protein: 0.6 g

Spicy Eggplant Cubes

Preparation Time: 10 minutes
Cooking Time: 20 minutes
Servings: 2
Ingredients:

- 12 oz. eggplants
- ½ tsp. cayenne pepper
- ½ tsp. ground black pepper
- ½ tsp. cilantro
- ½ tsp. ground paprika

Directions:

1. Rinse the eggplants and slice them into cubes.
2. Sprinkle the eggplant cubes with the cayenne pepper and ground black pepper.
3. Add the cilantro and ground paprika.
4. Stir the mixture well and let it rest for 10 minutes.
5. After this, sprinkle the eggplants with olive oil and place in the air fry basket.
6. Cook the eggplants for 20 minutes at 380°F, stirring halfway through.
7. When the eggplant cubes are done, serve them right away!

Nutrition:

- Calories: 67
- Fats: 2.8 g
- Fiber: 6.5 g
- Carbs: 10.9 g
- Protein: 1.9 g

Roasted Garlic Head

Preparation Time: 5 minutes
Cooking Time: 10 minutes

Servings: 4
Ingredients:

- 1 lb. garlic head
- 1 tbsp. olive oil
- 1 tsp. thyme

Directions:
1. Cut the ends of the garlic head and place it in the air fry basket.
2. Then sprinkle the garlic head with the olive oil and thyme.
3. Cook the garlic head for 10 minutes at 400°F.
4. When the garlic head is cooked, it should be soft and aromatic.
5. Serve immediately.

Nutrition:

- Calories: 200
- Fats: 4.1 g
- Fiber: 2.5 g
- Carbs: 37.7 g
- Protein: 7.2 g

Wrapped Asparagus

Preparation Time: 10 minutes
Cooking Time: 5 minutes
Servings: 4
Ingredients:

- 12 oz. asparagus
- ½ tsp. ground black pepper
- 3 oz. turkey fillet, sliced
- ¼ tsp. chili flakes

Directions:
1. Sprinkle the asparagus with the ground black pepper and chili flakes.
2. Stir carefully.
3. Wrap the asparagus in the sliced turkey fillet and place in the air fry basket.
4. Cook the asparagus at 400°F for 5 minutes, turning halfway through cooking.
5. Let the wrapped asparagus cool for 2 minutes before serving.

Nutrition:

- Calories: 133
- Fats: 9 g
- Fiber: 1.9 g
- Carbs: 3.8 g
- Protein: 9.8 g

Baked Yams with Dill

Preparation Time: 10 minutes
Cooking Time: 8 minutes
Servings: 2
Ingredients:

- 2 yams
- 1 tbsp. fresh dill
- 1 tsp. coconut oil
- ½ tsp. minced garlic

Directions:

- Wash the yams carefully and cut them into halves.
- Sprinkle the yam halves with the coconut oil and then rub with the minced garlic.
- Place the yams in the air fry basket and cook for 8 minutes at 400°F.
- After this, mash the yams gently with a fork and then sprinkle with the fresh dill.
- Serve the yams immediately.

Nutrition:

- Calories: 25
- Fats: 2.3 g
- Fiber: 0.2 g
- Carbs: 1.2 g
- Protein: 0.4 g

Honey Onions

Preparation Time: 10 minutes
Cooking Time: 20 minutes
Servings: 2
Ingredients:

- 2 white onions, large
- 1 tbsp. raw honey
- 1 tsp. water
- 1 tbsp. paprika

Directions:
1. Peel the onions, and using a knife, make cuts in the shape of a cross.
2. Then combine the raw honey and water; stir.
3. Add the paprika and stir the mixture until smooth.
4. Place the onions in the air fryer basket and sprinkle them with the honey mixture.
5. Cook the onions for 16 minutes at 380°F.

6. When the onions are cooked, they should be soft.

7. Transfer the cooked onions to serving plates and serve.

Nutrition:
- Calories: 10
- Fats: 0.6 g
- Fiber: 4.5 g
- Carbs: 24.6 g
- Protein: 2.2 g

Delightful Roasted Garlic Slices

Preparation Time: 10 minutes
Cooking Time: 8 minutes
Servings: 4
Ingredients:
- 1 tsp. coconut oil
- ½ tsp. cilantro, dried
- ¼ tsp. cayenne pepper
- 12 oz. garlic cloves, peeled

Directions:
1. Sprinkle the garlic cloves with the cayenne pepper and the dried cilantro.
2. Mix the garlic up with the spices, and then transfer to the air fry basket.
3. Add the coconut oil and cook the garlic for 8 minutes at 400°F, stirring halfway through.
4. When the garlic cloves are done, transfer them to serving plates and serve.

Nutrition:
- Calories: 137
- Fats: 1.6 g
- Fiber: 1.8 g
- Carbs: 28.2 g
- Protein: 5.4 g

Coconut Oil Artichokes

Preparation Time: 10 minutes
Cooking Time: 13 minutes
Servings: 4
Ingredients:
- 1 lb. artichokes
- 1 tbsp. coconut oil
- 1 tbsp. water
- ½ tsp. minced garlic
- ¼ tsp. cayenne pepper

Directions:

1. Trim the ends of the artichokes, sprinkle them with the water, and rub them with the minced garlic.
2. Sprinkle with the cayenne pepper and the coconut oil.
3. After this, wrap the artichokes in foil and place in the air fryer basket.
4. Cook for 10 minutes at 370°F.
5. Then remove the artichokes from the foil and cook them for 3 minutes more at 400°F.
6. Transfer the cooked artichokes to serving plates and let them cool a little.
7. Serve!

Nutrition:
- Calories: 83
- Fats: 3.6 g
- Fiber: 6.2 g
- Carbs: 12.1 g
- Protein: 3.7 g

Roasted Mushrooms

Preparation Time: 10 minutes
Cooking Time: 5 minutes
Servings: 2
Ingredients:
- 12 oz. mushroom hats
- ¼ cup fresh dill, chopped
- ¼ tsp. onion, chopped
- 1 tsp. olive oil
- ¼ tsp. turmeric

Directions:
1. Combine the chopped dill and onion.
2. Add the turmeric and stir the mixture.
3. After this, add the olive oil and mix until homogenous.
4. Then fill the mushroom hats with the dill mixture and place them in the air fry basket.
5. Cook the mushrooms for 5 minutes at 400°F.
6. When the vegetables are cooked, let them cool to room temperature before serving.

Nutrition:
- Calories: 73
- Fats: 3.1 g
- Fiber: 2.6 g
- Carbs: 9.2 g
- Protein: 6.6 g

Mashed Yams

Preparation Time: 10 minutes
Cooking Time: 10 minutes
Servings: 5
Ingredients:
- 1 lb. yams
- 1 tsp. olive oil
- 1 tbsp. almond milk
- ¾ tsp. salt
- 1 tsp. dried parsley

Directions:
1. Peel the yams and chop them.
2. Place the chopped yams in the air fry basket and sprinkle with the salt and dried parsley.
3. Add the olive oil and stir the mixture.
4. Cook the yams at 400°F for 10 minutes, stirring twice during cooking.
5. When the yams are done, blend them well with a hand blender until smooth.
6. Add the almond milk and stir carefully.
7. Serve, and enjoy!

Nutrition:
- Calories: 120
- Fats: 1.8 g
- Fiber: 3.6 g
- Carbs: 25.1 g
- Protein: 1.4 g

Cauliflower Rice

Preparation Time: 10 minutes
Cooking Time: 12 minutes
Servings: 4
Ingredients:
- 14 oz. cauliflower heads
- 1 tbsp. coconut oil
- 2 tbsp. fresh parsley, chopped

Directions:
1. Wash the cauliflower heads carefully and chop them into small pieces of rice.
2. Place the cauliflower in the air fry and add coconut oil.
3. Stir carefully and cook for 10 minutes at 370°F.
4. Then add the fresh parsley and stir well.
5. Cook the cauliflower rice for 2 minutes more at 400°F.

6. After this, gently toss the cauliflower rice and serve immediately.

Nutrition:
- Calories: 55
- Fats: 3.5 g
- Fiber: 2.5 g
- Carbs: 5.4 g
- Protein: 2 g

Shredded Cabbage

Preparation Time: 15 minutes
Cooking Time: 15 minutes
Servings: 4
Ingredients:
- 15 oz. cabbage
- ¼ tsp. salt
- ¼ cup chicken stock
- ½ tsp. paprika

Directions:
1. Shred the cabbage and sprinkle it with the salt and paprika.
2. Stir the cabbage and let it sit for 10 minutes.
3. Then transfer the cabbage to the air fry basket and add the chicken stock.
4. Cook the cabbage for 15 minutes at 250°F, stirring halfway through.
5. When the cabbage is soft, it is done.
6. Serve immediately, while still hot.

Nutrition:
- Calories: 132
- Fats: 2.1 g
- Carbs: 32.1 g
- Protein: 1.78 g

Fried Leeks Recipe

Preparation Time: 5 minutes
Cooking Time: 10 minutes
Servings: 4
Ingredients:
- 4 leeks; ends cut off and halved
- 1 tbsp. butter; melted
- 1 tbsp. lemon juice
- Salt and black pepper to taste

Directions:
- Coat the leeks with the melted butter, flavor with salt and black pepper, put in your Air Fry Oven and cook at 350°F, for 7 minutes.

- Arrange on a platter, drizzle the lemon juice all over and serve.

Nutrition:
- Calories: 100
- Fats: 4 g
- Fiber: 2 g
- Carbs: 6 g
- Protein: 2 g

Brussels Sprouts and Tomatoes Mix Recipe

Preparation Time: 5 minutes
Cooking Time: 10 minutes
Servings: 4
Ingredients:
- 1 lb. Brussels sprouts; trimmed
- 6 cherry tomatoes; halved
- ¼ cup green onions; chopped.
- 1 tbsp. olive oil
- Salt and black pepper to the taste

Directions:
1. Season Brussels sprouts with salt and pepper, put them in your Air Fry Oven and cook at 350°F for 10 minutes.
2. Transfer them to a bowl, add the salt, pepper, cherry tomatoes, green onions and olive oil, toss well and serve.

Nutrition:
- Calories: 121
- Fats: 4 g
- Fiber: 4 g
- Carbs: 11 g
- Protein: 4 g

Radish Hash Recipe

Preparation Time: 5 minutes
Cooking Time: 15 minutes
Servings: 4
Ingredients:
- ½ tsp. onion powder
- ⅓ cup parmesan, grated
- 4 eggs
- 1 lb. radishes, sliced
- Salt and black pepper to taste

Directions:
1. In a bowl; mix the radishes with salt, pepper, onion, eggs and parmesan and stir well.

2. Transfer the radishes to a pan that fits your air fryer and cook at 350°F for 7 minutes.
3. Divide the hash on plates and serve.

Nutrition:
- Calories: 80
- Fats: 5 g
- Fiber: 2 g
- Carbs: 5 g
- Protein: 7 g

Broccoli Salad Recipe

Preparation Time: 5 minutes
Cooking Time: 20 minutes
Servings: 4
Ingredients:
- 1 broccoli head, florets separated
- 1 tbsp. Chinese rice wine vinegar
- 1 tbsp. peanut oil
- 6 garlic cloves, minced
- Salt and black pepper to taste

Directions:
1. In a bowl, mix broccoli with salt, pepper and half of the oil, toss, transfer to your Air Fry Oven and cook at 350°F for 8 minutes, shaking the fryer halfway
2. Transfer the broccoli to a salad bowl, add the rest of the peanut oil, garlic and rice vinegar, toss really well and serve.

Nutrition:
- Calories: 121
- Fats: 3 g
- Fiber: 4 g
- Carbs: 4 g
- Protein: 4 g

Chili Broccoli

Preparation Time: 5 minutes
Cooking Time: 15 minutes
Servings: 4
Ingredients:
- 1-lb. broccoli florets
- 2 tbsp. olive oil
- 2 tbsp. chili sauce
- Juice of 1 lime
- A pinch of salt and black pepper

Directions:

1. Combine all of the ingredients in a bowl, and toss well.
2. Put the broccoli in your air fryer's basket and cook at 400 degrees F for 15 minutes.
3. Divide between plates and serve.

Nutrition:
- Calories: 173
- Fats: 6 g
- Fiber: 2 g
- Carbs: 6 g
- Protein: 8 g

Parmesan Broccoli and Asparagus

Preparation Time: 5 minutes
Cooking Time: 15 minutes
Servings: 4
Ingredients:
- 1 broccoli head, florets separated
- ½ lb. asparagus, trimmed
- Juice of 1 lime
- Salt and black pepper to the taste
- 2 tbsp. olive oil
- 3 tbsp. parmesan, grated

Directions:
1. In a small bowl, combine the asparagus with the broccoli and all the other ingredients except the parmesan, toss, transfer to your air fry basket and cook at 400ºF for 15 minutes.
2. Divide between plates, sprinkle the parmesan on top and serve.

Nutrition:
- Calories: 172
- Fats: 5 g
- Fiber: 2 g
- Carbs: 4 g
- Protein: 9 g

Butter Broccoli Mix

Preparation Time: 5 minutes
Cooking Time: 15 minutes
Servings: 4
Ingredients:
- 1 lb. broccoli florets
- A pinch of salt and black pepper
- 1 tsp. sweet paprika
- ½ tbsp. butter, melted

Directions:

1. In a small bowl, combine the broccoli with the rest of the ingredients, and toss.
2. Put the broccoli in your air fry basket, cook at 350ºF for 15 minutes, divide between plates and serve.

Nutrition:
- Calories: 130
- Fats: 3 g
- Fiber: 3 g
- Carbs: 4 g
- Protein: 8 g

Balsamic Kale

Preparation Time: 2 minutes
Cooking Time: 12 minutes
Servings: 6
Ingredients:
- 2 tbsp. olive oil
- 3 garlic cloves, minced
- 2 ½ lb. kale leaves
- Salt and black pepper to taste
- 2 tbsp. balsamic vinegar

Directions:
1. In a pan that fits the Air Fry Oven, combine all the ingredients and toss.
2. Put the pan in your Air Fry Ovenand cook at 300ºF for 12 minutes.
3. Divide between plates and serve.

Nutrition:
- Calories: 122
- Fats: 4 g
- Fiber: 3 g
- Carbs: 4 g
- Protein: 5 g

Kale and Olives

Preparation Time: 5 minutes
Cooking Time: 15 minutes
Servings: 4
Ingredients:
- 1 ½ lb. kale, torn
- 2 tbsp. olive oil
- Salt and black pepper to taste
- 1 tbsp. hot paprika
- 2 tbsp. black olives, pitted and sliced

Directions:

1. In a pan that fits the Air Fry, combine all the ingredients and toss.
2. Put the pan in your Air Fry, cook at 370ºF for 15 minutes, divide between plates and serve.

Nutrition:
- Calories: 154
- Fats: 3 g
- Fiber: 2 g
- Carbs: 4 g
- Protein: 6 g

Kale and Mushrooms Mix

Preparation Time: 5 minutes
Cooking Time: 15 minutes
Servings: 4
Ingredients:
- 1 lb. brown mushrooms, sliced
- 1 lb. kale, torn
- Salt and black pepper to the taste
- 2 tbsp. olive oil
- 14 oz. coconut milk

Directions:
1. In a pot that fits your Air Fry Oven, mix the kale with the rest of the ingredients and toss.
2. Put the pan in the fryer, cook at 380ºF for 15 minutes, divide between plates and serve.

Nutrition:
- Calories: 162
- Fats: 4 g
- Fiber: 1 g
- Carbs: 3 g
- Protein: 5 g

Oregano Kale

Preparation Time: 5 minutes
Cooking Time: 10 minutes
Servings: 4
Ingredients:
- 1 lb. kale, torn
- 1 tbsp. olive oil
- A pinch of salt and black pepper
- 2 tbsp. oregano, chopped

Directions:
1. In a pan that fits the Air Fry Oven, combine all the ingredients and toss.
2. Put the pan in the air fryer and cook at 380ºF for 10 minutes.
3. Divide between plates and serve.

Nutrition:
- Calories: 140
- Fats: 3 g
- Fiber: 2 g
- Carbs: 3 g
- Protein: 5 g

Kale and Brussels Sprouts

Preparation Time: 5 minutes
Cooking Time: 15 minutes
Servings: 8
Ingredients:
- 1 lb. Brussels sprouts, trimmed
- 2 cups kale, torn
- 1 tbsp. olive oil
- Salt and black pepper to taste
- 3 oz. mozzarella, shredded

Directions:
1. In a pan that fits the Air Fry Oven, combine all the ingredients except the mozzarella and toss.
2. Put the pan in the Air Fry Oven and cook at 380ºF for 15 minutes.
3. Divide between plates, sprinkle the cheese on top and serve.

Nutrition:
- Calories: 170
- Fats: 5 g
- Fiber: 3 g
- Carbs: 4 g
- Protein: 7 g

CHAPTER 7: SEAFOOD

Breaded Coconut Shrimp

Preparation Time: 5 minutes
Cooking Time: 15 minutes
Servings: 4
Ingredients:

- 1 lb. shrimp
- 1 cup panko breadcrumbs
- 1 cup coconut, shredded
- 2 eggs
- ⅓ cup all-purpose flour

Directions:

1. Fix the temperature of the Air Fryer at 360º Fahrenheit.
2. Peel and devein the shrimp.
3. Whisk the seasonings with the flour as desired. In another bowl, whisk the eggs, and in the third bowl, combine the breadcrumbs and coconut.
4. Dip the cleaned shrimp into the flour, egg wash, and finish it off with the coconut mixture.
5. Lightly, spray the basket of the Air Fry Oven and set the timer for 10–15 minutes.
6. Air-fry until it's a golden brown before serving.

Nutrition:

- Calories: 285
- Fats: 12.8 g
- Carbs: 3.7 g
- Protein: 38.1 g

Breaded Cod Sticks

Preparation Time: 5 minutes
Cooking Time: 20 minutes
Servings: 4
Ingredients:

- 2 large eggs
- 3 tbsp. milk
- 2 cups breadcrumbs
- 1 cups almond flour
- 1 lb. cod

Directions:

1. Heat the Air Fry Oven to 350ºF.
2. Prepare 3 bowls; one with the milk and eggs, one with the breadcrumbs (salt and pepper if desired), and another with almond flour.
3. Dip the sticks in the flour, egg mixture, and breadcrumbs.
4. Place in the basket and set the timer for 12 minutes. Toss the basket halfway through the cooking process.
5. Serve with your favorite sauce.

Nutrition:

- Calories: 254
- Fats: 14.2 g
- Carbs: 5.7 g
- Protein: 39.1 g

Cajun Shrimp

Preparation Time: 5 minutes
Cooking Time: 5 minutes
Servings: 6
Ingredients:

- 16–20 (1 ¼-lb.) tiger shrimp
- 1 tbsp. olive oil
- .5 tsp. OLD BAY® seasoning
- .25 tsp. smoked paprika
- .25 tsp. cayenne pepper

Directions:

1. Set the Air Fry Oven to 390º Fahrenheit.
2. Cover the shrimp using the oil and spices.
3. Toss them into the Air Fry basket and set the timer for 5 minutes.
4. Serve with your favorite side dish.

Nutrition:

- Calories: 356
- Fats: 18 g
- Carbs: 5 g
- Protein: 34 g

Cod Fish Nuggets

Preparation Time: 5 minutes
Cooking Time: 20 minutes
Servings: 4
Ingredients:

- 1 lb. cod fillet
- 3 eggs
- 4 tbsp. olive oil
- 1 cup almond flour
- 1 cup breadcrumbs, gluten-free

Directions:

1. Heat the Air Fry Oven to 390ºF.
2. Slice the cod into nuggets.
3. Prepare 3 bowls and whisk the eggs in one of them. Combine the salt, oil, and breadcrumbs in another bowl. Sift the almond flour into the third bowl.
4. Cover each of the nuggets with the flour, dip in the eggs, and the breadcrumbs.
5. Arrange the nuggets in the basket and set the timer for 20 minutes.
6. Serve the fish with your favorite dips or sides.

Nutrition:
- Calories: 334
- Fats: 10 g
- Carbs: 8 g
- Protein: 32 g

Creamy Salmon

Preparation Time: 5 minutes
Cooking Time: 20 minutes
Servings: 4
Ingredients:
- 1 tbsp. dill, chopped
- 1 tbsp. olive oil
- 1 ¾ oz. plain yogurt
- 6 pieces (¾-lb.) salmon

Directions:
1. Heat the Air Fry Oven and wait for it to reach 285ºF.
2. Shake the salt over the salmon and add them to the fryer basket with the olive oil to air-fry for 10 minutes.
3. Whisk the yogurt, salt, and dill.
4. Serve the salmon with the sauce or side dish of your preference.

Nutrition:
- Calories: 340
- Carbs: 5 g
- Fats: 16 g
- Protein: 32 g

Crumbled Fish

Preparation Time: 5 minutes
Cooking Time: 15 minutes
Servings: 4
Ingredients:

- .5 cup breadcrumbs
- 4 tbsp. vegetable oil
- 1 egg
- 4 fish fillets
- 1 lemon

Directions:
1. Heat the Air Fry Oven to 356ºF.
2. Whisk the oil and breadcrumbs until crumbly.
3. Dip the fish into the egg, then in the crumb mixture.
4. Arrange the fish fillets in the Air Fry Oven and air-fry for 12 minutes.
5. Garnish with the lemon.

Nutrition:
- Calories: 320
- Carbs: 8 g
- Fats: 10 g
- Protein: 28 g

Easy Crab Sticks

Preparation Time: 5 minutes
Cooking Time: 10 minutes
Servings: 4
Ingredients:
- 1 package crab sticks
- Cooking oil spray as needed

Directions:
1. Take each of the sticks out of the package and unroll it until the sticks are flat. Tear the sheets into thirds.
2. Arrange them on the air fryer basket and spray lightly with the cooking oil. Set the timer for 10 minutes.

Tip: If you shred the crab meat, you can cut the time in half, but they will also easily fall through the holes in the basket.

Nutrition:
- Calories: 285
- Fats: 12.8 g
- Carbs: 3.7 g
- Protein: 38.1 g

Fried Catfish

Preparation Time: 5 minutes
Cooking Time: 15 minutes
Servings: 4

Ingredients:
- 1 tbsp. olive oil
- .25 cup seasoned fish fry
- 4 catfish fillets

Directions:
1. Heat the Air Fry Oven to 400ºFbefore 'fry' time.
2. Rinse the catfish and pat dry using a paper towel.
3. Dump the seasoning into a sizeable Ziploc® bag. Add the fish and shake to cover each fillet. Spray with the cooking oil spray and add to the basket.
4. Set the timer for 10 minutes. Flip, and reset the timer for ten additional minutes. Turn the fish once more and cook for 2–3 minutes.
5. Once it reaches the desired crispiness, transfer to a plate and serve.

Nutrition:
- Calories: 376
- Fats: 9 g
- Carbs: 10 g
- Protein: 28 g

Grilled Sardines

Preparation Time: 5 minutes
Cooking Time: 20 minutes
Servings: 4
Ingredients:
- 5 sardines

Directions:
1. Preheat the Air Fry Oven to 320ºF.
2. Place the sardines in the air fry basket.
3. Set the timer to 14 minutes. After 7 minutes, remember to turn the sardines so that they are roasted on both sides.

Nutrition:
- Calories: 189 g
- Fats: 10 g
- Protein: 22 g
- Cholesterol: 128 mg

Zucchini with Tuna

Preparation Time: 10 minutes
Cooking Time: 30 minutes
Servings: 4
Ingredients:
- 4 medium zucchinis
- 4 1/5 oz. tuna in oil (canned) drained
- 1 oz. grated cheese
- 1 tsp. pine nuts
- Salt, pepper to taste

Directions:
1. Cut the zucchini in half, laterally, and empty it with a small spoon (set aside the pulp that will be used for filling); place them in the basket.
2. In a food processor, put the zucchini pulp, drained tuna, pine nuts and grated cheese. Mix everything until you get a homogeneous and dense mixture.
3. Fill the zucchini. Set the Air Fry Oven to 356ºF.
4. Simmer for 20 min, depending on the size of the zucchini. Let cool before serving.

Nutrition:
- Calories: 389
- Carbs: 10 g
- Fats: 29 g
- Sugar: 5 g
- Protein: 23 g
- Cholesterol: 40 mg

Caramelized Salmon Fillet

Preparation Time: 5 minutes
Cooking Time: 25 minutes
Servings: 4
Ingredients:
- 2 salmon fillets
- 2 oz. cane sugar
- 4 tbsp. soy sauce
- 1 ¾450g sesame seeds
- Fresh ginger

Directions:
1. Preheat the Air Fry Oven at 356ºF for 5 minutes.
2. Put the cane sugar and soy sauce in the basket.
3. Cook everything for 5 minutes.
4. In the meantime, wash the salmon fillets well, pass it through the sesame seeds to cover it completely and place it inside the tank and add the fresh ginger.
5. Cook for 12 minutes.
6. Turn the fish over and finish cooking for another 8 minutes.

Nutrition:
- Calories: 569
- Fats: 14.9 g
- Carbs: 40 g
- Sugar: 27.6 g
- Protein: 66.9 g
- Cholesterol: 165.3 mg

Deep Fried Prawns

Preparation Time: 15 minutes
Cooking Time: 20 minutes
Servings: 6
Ingredients:
- 12 prawns
- 2 eggs
- ½ tsp. Flour to taste
- 1 tbsp Breadcrumbs
- 4 tbsp Yogurt
- 2 tbsp Mayonnaise sauce

Directions:
1. Remove the head of the prawns and shell carefully.
2. Dip the prawns first in the flour, then in the beaten eggs and then in the breadcrumbs.
3. Preheat the Air Fry Oven for 1 minute at 302ºF.
4. Add the prawns and cook for 4 minutes. If the prawns are large, it will be necessary to cook 6 at a time.
5. Turn the prawns and cook for another 4 minutes.
6. They should be served with a yogurt or mayonnaise sauce.

Nutrition:
- Calories: 2385.1
- Fats: 23
- Carbs: 52.3 g
- Sugar: 0.1 g
- Protein: 21.4 g

Mussels with Pepper

Preparation Time: 15 minutes
Cooking Time: 20 minutes
Servings: 5
Ingredients:
- 1 ½ lb. mussels
- 1 clove garlic
- 1 tsp. oil
- ½ tsp. Pepper to taste
- ½ tsp. Parsley Taste

Directions:
1. Clean and scrape the mussels cover and remove the byssus (the "beard" that comes out of the mussels.)
2. Pour the oil, clean the mussels and the crushed garlic in the air fryer basket. Set the temperature to 392ºF and simmer for 12 minutes. Towards the end of cooking, add the black pepper and the chopped parsley.
3. Finally, distribute the mussel juice well at the bottom of the basket, shaking the basket.

Nutrition:
- Calories: 150
- Carbs: 2 g
- Fats: 8 g
- Protein: 15 g

Monkfish with Olives and Capers

Preparation Time: 25 minutes
Cooking Time: 40 minutes
Servings: 4
Ingredients:
- 1 monkfish
- 10 cherry tomatoes
- 1 ¾ cailletier olives
- 5 capers

Directions:
1. Spread aluminum foil inside the air fry basket and place the monkfish clean and skinless.
2. Chop the tomatoes and add them with the olives, capers, oil, and salt.
3. Set the temperature to 320ºF.
4. Cook the monkfish for about 40 minutes.

Nutrition:
- Calories: 404
- Fats: 29 g
- Carbs: 36 g
- Sugar: 7 g
- Protein: 24 g
- Cholesterol: 36 mg

Shrimp, Zucchini and Cherry Tomato Sauce

Preparation Time: 5 minutes

Cooking Time: 30 minutes
Servings: 4
Ingredients:

- 2 zucchinis
- 300 shrimps
- 7 cherry tomatoes
- Salt and pepper to taste
- 1 garlic clove

Directions:

1. Pour the oil in the Air Fry Oven, and add the garlic clove and diced zucchini.
2. Cook for 15 minutes at 302ºF.
3. Add the shrimps and the tomato pieces, salt, and spices.
4. Cook for another 5–10 minutes or until the shrimp water evaporates.

Nutrition:

- Calories: 214.3
- Fats: 8.6 g
- Carbs: 7.8 g
- Sugar: 4.8 g
- Protein: 27.0 g
- Cholesterol: 232.7 mg

Salmon with Pistachio Bark

Preparation Time: 10 minutes
Cooking Time: 30 minutes
Servings: 4
Ingredients:

- 1 ⅓ lb. salmon fillet
- 1 ⅓ oz. pistachios
- Salt to taste

Directions:

1. Put the parchment paper on the bottom of the air fryer basket and place the salmon fillet in it (it can be cooked whole or already divided into four portions).
2. Cut the pistachios in thick pieces, grease the top of the fish, and salt (little because the pistachios are already salted), and cover everything with the pistachios.
3. Set the air fryer to 356ºF and simmer for 25 minutes.

Nutrition:

- Calories: 371.7
- Fats: 21.8 g
- Carbs: 9.4 g

- Sugar: 2.2 g
- Protein: 34.7 g
- Cholesterol: 80.5 mg

Salted Marinated Salmon

Preparation Time: 10 minutes
Cooking Time: 30 minutes
Servings: 4
Ingredients:

- 1 lb. salmon fillet
- 16 lb. coarse salt
- 1 tbsp Oil

Directions:

1. Place some baking paper on the air fry basket and the salmon on top (skin-side up) covered with coarse salt.
2. Set the air fryer to 302ºF.
3. Cook everything for 25–30 minutes. At the end of cooking, remove the fish and serve with a drizzle of oil.

Nutrition:

- Calories: 290
- Fats: 13 g
- Carbs: 3 g
- Protein: 40 g
- Cholesterol: 196 mg

Sautéed Trout with Almonds

Preparation Time: 35 minutes
Cooking Time: 20 minutes
Servings: 4
Ingredients:

- 1 1/5 lb. salmon trout
- 15 black peppercorns
- 2 Dill leaves to taste
- 1 oz. almonds
- ½ tsp. Salt to taste
- 1 tbsp Oil

Directions:

1. Cut the trout into cubes and marinate it for half an hour with the rest of the ingredients (except salt).
2. Cook in air fryer for 17 minutes at 320ºF. Drizzle with oil and salt and serve.

Nutrition:

- Calories: 238.5
- Fats: 20.1 g

- Carbs: 11.5 g
- Sugar: 1.0 g
- Protein: 4.0 g
- Cholesterol: 45.9 mg

Calamari Slices

Preparation Time: 5 minutes
Cooking Time: 12 minutes
Servings: 4
Ingredients:

- 16 calamari slices
- 1 egg
- 1 tbsp Breadcrumbs
- ½ tsp. Salt, pepper, sweet paprika

Directions:

1. Put the calamari slices in the air fryer to boil for 2 minutes.
2. Remove and dry them well.
3. Beat the egg and season to taste. Add the egg mixture to the calamari slices and serve with the breadcrumbs.

Nutrition:

- Calories: 356
- Fats: 18 g
- Carbs: 5 g
- Protein: 34 g

Honey Glazed Salmon

Preparation Time: 10 minutes
Cooking Time: 8 minutes
Servings: 2
Ingredients:

- 2 (6-oz.) salmon fillets
- ½ tsp. Salt, as required
- 2 tbsp. honey

Directions:

1. Sprinkle the salmon fillets with salt and then, coat with honey.
2. Press the "Power" button of the Air Fry Oven and turn the dial to select the "Air Fry" mode.
3. Press the "Time" button and again turn the dial to set the cooking time to 8 minutes.
4. Now push the "Temp" button and rotate the dial to set the temperature at 355ºF.
5. Press the "Start/Pause" button to start.
6. Open the unit when it is already hot, when it beeps.

7. Arrange the salmon fillets in a greased air fry basket and insert them in the Air Fry Oven.
8. Serve hot.

Nutrition:

- Calories: 289
- Fats: 10.5 g
- Carbs: 17.3 g
- Protein: 33.1 g

Sweet & Sour Glazed Salmon

Preparation Time: 12 minutes
Cooking Time: 20 minutes
Servings: 2
Ingredients:

- ⅓ cup soy sauce
- ⅓ cup honey
- 3 tsp. rice wine vinegar
- 1 tsp. water
- 4 (3 ½-oz.) salmon fillets

Directions:

1. Mix the soy sauce, honey, vinegar, and water together in a bowl.
2. In another small bowl, reserve about half of the mixture.
3. Add the salmon fillets in the remaining mixture and coat them well.
4. Cover the bowl and refrigerate to marinate for about 2 hours.
5. Press the "Power" button of the Air Fry Oven and turn the dial to select the "Air Fry" mode.
6. Press the "Time" button and again turn the dial to set the cooking time to 12 minutes.
7. Now push the "Temp" button and rotate the dial to set the temperature at 355ºF.
8. Press the "Start/Pause" button to start.
9. Open the unit when it is already hot, when it beeps.
10. Arrange the salmon fillets in greased air fry basket" and insert them in the Air Fry Oven.
11. Flip the salmon fillets once halfway through and coat them with the reserved marinade after every 3 minutes.
12. Serve hot.

Nutrition:

- Calories: 462
- Fats: 12.3 g
- Carbs: 49.8 g

- Protein: 41.3 g

Ranch Tilapia

Preparation Time: 15 minutes
Cooking Time: 13 minutes
Servings: 4
Ingredients:

- ¾ cup cornflakes, crushed
- 1 (1-oz.) packet dry ranch-style dressing mix
- 2 ½ tbsp. vegetable oil
- 2 eggs
- 4 (6-oz.) tilapia fillets

Directions:

1. In a shallow bowl, beat the eggs.
2. In another bowl, add the cornflakes, ranch dressing, and oil and mix until a crumbly mixture form.
3. Dip the tilapia fillets into the egg mixture and then, and coat them with the bread crumbs mixture.
4. Press the "Power" button of the Air Fry Oven and turn the dial to select the "Air Fry" mode.
5. Press the "Time" button and again turn the dial to set the cooking time to 13 minutes.
6. Now push the "Temp" button and rotate the dial to set the temperature at 356ºF.
7. Press the "Start/Pause" button to start.
8. Open the unit when it is already hot, when it beeps.
9. Arrange the tilapia fillets in greased air fry basket and insert them in the Air Fry Oven.
10. Serve hot.

Nutrition:

- Calories: 267
- Fats: 12.2 g
- Carbs: 5.1 g
- Protein: 34.9 g

Breaded Flounder

Preparation Time: 15 minutes
Cooking Time: 12 minutes
Servings: 3
Ingredients:

- 1 egg
- 1 cup dry breadcrumbs
- ¼ cup vegetable oil

- 3 (6-oz.) flounder fillets
- 1 lemon, sliced

Directions:

1. In a shallow bowl, beat the egg.

Don't capitalize	Use double quotation

2. In another bowl, add the breadcrumbs and oil and mix until the crumbly mixture is formed.
3. Dip the flounder fillets into the beaten egg and then coat with the breadcrumb mixture.
4. Press the "Power" button of the Air Fry Oven and turn the dial to select the "Air Fry" mode.
5. Press the "Time" button and again turn the dial to set the cooking time to 12 minutes.
6. Now push the "Temp" button and rotate the dial to set the temperature at 356ºF.
7. Press the "Start/Pause" button to start.
8. Open the unit when it is already hot, when it beeps.
9. Arrange the flounder fillets in a greased air fry basket and insert them in the Air Fry Oven.
10. Plate with lemon slices and serve hot.

Nutrition:

- Calories: 524
- Fats: 24.2 g
- Saturated Fats: 5.1 g
- Cholesterol: 170 mg
- Sodium: 463 mg
- Carbs: 26.5 g
- Fiber: 1.5 g
- Sugar: 2.5 g
- Protein: 47.8 g

Simple Haddock

Preparation Time: 15 minutes
Cooking Time: 8 minutes
Servings: 2
Ingredients:

- 2 (6-oz.) haddock fillets
- 1 tbsp. olive oil
- Salt and ground black pepper, as required

Directions:

1. Coat the haddock fillets with oil and then sprinkle with salt and black pepper.
2. Press the "Power" button of the Air Fry Oven and turn the dial to select the "Air Fry" mode.

3. Press the "Time" button and again turn the dial to set the cooking time to 8 minutes.

4. Now push the "Temp" button and rotate the dial to set the temperature at 355ºF.

5. Press the "Start/Pause" button to start.

6. Open the unit when it is already hot, when it beeps.

7. Arrange the haddock fillets in a greased air fry basket and insert them in the Air Fry Oven.

8. Serve hot.

Nutrition:

- Calories: 251
- Fats: 8.6 g
- Saturated Fats: 1.3 g
- Cholesterol: 126 mg
- Sodium 226: mg
- Protein: 41.2 g

Breaded Hake

Preparation Time: 15 minutes
Cooking Time: 12 minutes
Servings: 4
Ingredients:

- 1 egg
- 4 oz. breadcrumbs
- 2 tbsp. vegetable oil
- 4 (6-oz.) hake fillets
- 1 lemon, cut into wedges

Directions:

1. Beat the egg in a large bowl.

2. In another bowl, add the breadcrumbs, and oil and mix until a crumbly mixture forms.

3. Dip hake fillets into the egg and then coat with the bread crumbs mixture.

4. Press the "Power" button of the Air Fry Oven and turn the dial to select the "Air Fry" mode.

5. Press the "Time" button and again turn the dial to set the cooking time to 12 minutes.

6. Now push the "Temp" button and rotate the dial to set the temperature at 350ºF.

7. Press the "Start/Pause" button to start.

8. Open the unit when it is already hot, when it beeps.

9. Arrange the hake fillets in a greased air fry basket and insert them in the Air Fry Oven.

10. Serve hot.

Nutrition:

- Calories: 297
- Fats: 10.6 g
- Saturated Fats: 2 g
- Cholesterol: 89 mg
- Sodium: 439 mg
- Carbs: 22 g
- Fiber: 1.4 g
- Sugar: 1.9 g
- Protein: 29.2 g

Sesame Seeds Coated Tuna

Preparation Time: 15 minutes
Cooking Time: 6 minutes
Servings: 2
Ingredients:

- 1 egg white
- ¼ cup white sesame seeds
- 1 tbsp. black sesame seeds
- Salt and ground black pepper, as required
- 2 (6-oz.) tuna steaks

Directions:

1. Beat the egg white in a large bowl.

2. In another bowl, mix together the sesame seeds, salt, and black pepper.

3. Dip the tuna steaks into the beaten egg white and then coat with the sesame seeds mixture.

4. Press the "Power" button of the Air Fry Oven and turn the dial to select the "Air Fry" mode.

5. Press the "Time" button and again turn the dial to set the cooking time to 6 minutes.

6. Now push the "Temp" button and rotate the dial to set the temperature at 400 degrees F.

7. Press the "Start/Pause" button to start.

8. Open the unit when it is already hot, when it beeps.

9. Arrange the tuna steaks in greased "Air Fry Basket" and insert them in the Air Fry Oven.

10. Flip the tuna steaks once halfway through.

11. Serve hot.

Nutrition:

- Calories: 450
- Total Fats: 21.9 g
- Saturated Fats: 4.3 g
- Cholesterol: 83 mg
- Sodium: 182 mg
- Carbs: 5.4 g
- Fiber: 2.7 g

- Sugar: 0.2 g
- Protein: 56.7 g

Cheese and Ham Patties

Preparation Time: 10 minutes
Cooking Time: 10 minutes
Servings: 4
Ingredients:
- 1 puff pastry sheet
- 4 handfuls mozzarella cheese, grated
- 4 tsp. mustard
- 8 ham slices, chopped

Directions:
1. Spread out the puff pastry on a clean surface and cut it into 12 squares.
2. Divide the cheese, ham, and mustard on half of them, top with the other halves, and seal the edges.
3. Place all the patties in your air fry basket and cook at 370ºF for 10 minutes.
4. Divide the patties between plates and serve.

Nutrition:
- Calories: 212
- Fats: 12 g
- Fiber: 7 g
- Carbs: 14 g
- Protein: 8 g

Air-Fried Seafood

Preparation Time: 10 minutes
Cooking Time: 10 minutes
Servings: 4
Ingredients:
- 1 lb. fresh scallops, mussels, fish fillets, prawns, shrimp
- 2 eggs, lightly beaten
- Salt and black pepper
- 1 cup breadcrumbs mixed with the zest of 1 lemon
- Cooking spray

Directions:
1. Clean the seafood as needed.
2. Dip each piece into the egg mixture and season with salt and pepper.
3. Coat the seafood in the crumbs and spray with oil.

4. Arrange the seafood in the Air Fry Oven and cook for 6 minutes at 400ºF. turning once halfway through.
5. Serve and Enjoy!

Nutrition:
- Calories: 133
- Protein: 17.4 g
- Fats: 3.1 g
- Carbs: 8.2 g

Fish with Chips

Preparation Time: 5 minutes
Cooking Time: 20 minutes
Servings: 2
Ingredients:
- 1 (6-oz.) cod fillet
- 3 cups salt
- 3 cups vinegar-flavored kettle cooked chips
- ¼ cup buttermilk
- Salt and pepper to taste

Directions:
1. Mix to combine the buttermilk, pepper, and salt in a bowl. Put the cod and leave to soak for 5 minutes
2. Put the chips in a food processor and process until crushed. Transfer the chips to a shallow bowl. Coat the fillet with the crushed chips.
3. Put the coated fillet in the air fry basket. Cook for 12 minutes at 400ºF.
4. Serve and Enjoy!

Nutrition:
- Calories: 646
- Protein: 41 g
- Fats: 33 g
- Carbs: 48 g

Crumbly Fishcakes

Preparation Time: 5 minutes
Cooking Time: 10 minutes
Servings: 4
Ingredients:
- 8 oz. salmon, cooked
- 1 ½ oz. potatoes, mashed
- A handful of parsley, chopped
- 1 lemon zest
- 1 ¾ oz. plain flour

Directions:

1.   Carefully, flake the salmon. In a bowl, mix the flaked salmon, zest, capers, dill, and mashed potatoes.

2.   Form small cakes using the mixture and dust the cakes with flour; refrigerate for 60 minutes.

3.   Preheat your Air Fry Oven to 350ºF. and cook the cakes for 7 minutes. Serve chilled.

Nutrition:
- Calories: 210
- Protein: 10 g
- Fats: 7 g
- Carbs: 25 g

Bacon Wrapped Shrimp

Preparation Time: 10 minutes
Cooking Time: 20 minutes
Servings: 4
Ingredients:
- 16 bacon slices, thin
- 16 pieces tiger shrimp, peeled and deveined

Directions:

1.   Wrap each shrimp with a slice of bacon. Put all the finished pieces in tray and chill for 20 minutes.

2.   Arrange the bacon-wrapped shrimp in the air frying basket. Cook for 7 minutes at 390ºF. Transfer to a plate lined with paper towels to drain before serving.

Nutrition:
- Calories: 436
- Protein: 32 g
- Fats: 41.01 g
- Carbs: 0.8 g

Crab Legs

Preparation Time: 10 minutes
Cooking Time: 10 minutes
Servings: 4
Ingredients:
- 3 lb. crab legs
- ¼ cup salted butter, melted and divided
- ½ lemon, juiced
- ¼ tsp. garlic powder

Directions:

1.   In a bowl, toss the crab legs and 2 tbsp. of the melted butter together. Place the crab legs in the air fry basket

2.   Cook at 400°F for 15 minutes, giving the basket a good shake halfway through.

3.   Combine the remaining butter with the lemon juice and garlic powder.

4.   Crack open the cooked crab legs and remove the meat. Serve with the butter dip on the side, and enjoy!

Nutrition:
- Calories: 272
- Fats: 19 g
- Fiber: 9 g
- Carbs: 18 g
- Protein: 12 g

Fish Sticks

Preparation Time: 5 minutes
Cooking Time: 10 minutes
Servings: 4
Ingredients:
- 1 lb. whitefish
- 2 tbsp. Dijon mustard
- ¼ cup mayonnaise
- 1 ½ cup pork rinds, finely ground
- ¾ tsp. Cajun seasoning

Directions:

1.   Place the whitefish on a tissue to dry it off, then cut it up into slices about 2 inches thick.

2.   In one bowl, combine the mustard and mayonnaise, and in another, the Cajun seasoning and pork rinds.

3.   Coat the fish firstly in the mayo-mustard mixture, then in the Cajun-pork rind mixture. Give each slice a shake to remove any surplus. Then place the fish sticks in the basket of the air flyer.

4.   Cook at 400°F for 5 minutes. Turn the fish sticks over and cook for another 5 minutes on the other side.

5.   Serve warm with a dipping sauce of your choice and enjoy.

Nutrition:
- Calories: 212
- Fats: 12 g
- Fiber: 7 g
- Carbs: 14 g
- Protein: 8 g

Crusty Pesto Salmon

Preparation Time: 5 minutes
Cooking Time: 10 minutes
Servings: 2
Ingredients:

- ¼ cup almonds, roughly chopped
- ¼ cup pesto
- 2 (4-oz.) salmon fillets
- 2 tbsp. unsalted butter, melted

Directions:

1. Mix the almonds and pesto together.
2. Place the salmon fillets in a round baking dish, roughly 6 inches in diameter.
3. Brush the fillets with butter, followed up by the pesto mixture, ensuring to coat both the top and bottom of the filets. Put the baking dish inside the Air Fry Oven.
4. Cook for 12 minutes at 390°F.
5. The salmon is ready when it flakes easily when prodded with a fork. Serve warm.

Nutrition:

- Calories: 354
- Fats: 21 g
- Carbs: 23 g
- Protein: 19 g

Salmon Patties

Preparation Time: 5 minutes
Cooking Time: 10 minutes
Servings: 4
Ingredients:

- 1 tsp. chili powder
- 2 tbsp. full-fat mayonnaise
- ¼ cup ground pork rinds
- 2 (5-oz.) pouches cooked pink salmon
- 1 egg

Directions:

1. Stir everything together to prepare the patty mixture. If the mixture is dry or falling apart, add in more pork rinds as necessary.
2. Take equal-sized amounts of the mixture to form 4 patties, before placing the patties in the air fry basket.
3. Cook at 400°F for 8 minutes.
4. Halfway through cooking, flip the patties over. Once they are crispy, serve with the toppings of your choice and enjoy.

Nutrition:

- Calories: 325
- Fats: 21 g
- Carbs: 18 g
- Protein: 29 g

Cajun Salmon

Preparation Time: 5 minutes
Cooking Time: 10 minutes
Servings: 4
Ingredients:

- 2 (4-oz) skinless salmon fillets
- 2 tbsp. unsalted butter, melted
- 1 pinch ground cayenne pepper
- 1 tsp. paprika
- ½ tsp. garlic pepper

Directions:

1. Using a brush, apply the butter to the salmon fillets.
2. Combine the other ingredients and massage this mixture into the fillets. Place the fish inside you're the Air Fry Oven.
3. Cook for seven minutes at 390°F.
4. When the salmon is ready, it should flake apart easily.
5. Enjoy with the sides of your choosing.

Nutrition:

- Calories: 383
- Fats: 12 g
- Carbs: 29 g
- Protein: 31 g

Buttery Cod

Preparation Time: 5 minutes
Cooking Time: 10 minutes
Servings: 4
Ingredients:

- 2 (4-oz.) cod fillets
- 2 tbsp. salted butter, melted
- 1 tsp. OLD BAY® seasoning
- ½ medium lemon, sliced

Directions:

1. Place the cod fillets in a dish.
2. Brush with melted butter, season with OLD BAY® and top with some lemon slices.
3. Wrap the fish in aluminum foil and put into your Air Fry Oven
4. Cook for 8 minutes at 350°F.

5. The cod is ready when it flakes easily. Serve hot.

Nutrition:
- Calories: 354
- Fats: 21 g
- Carbs: 23 g
- Protein: 19 g

Sesame Tuna Steak

Preparation Time: 5 minutes
Cooking Time: 10 minutes
Servings: 4
Ingredients:
- 1 tbsp. coconut oil, melted
- 2 (6-oz.) tuna steaks
- ½ tsp. garlic powder
- 2 tsp. black sesame seeds
- 2 tsp. white sesame seeds

Directions:
1. Apply the coconut oil to the tuna steaks with a brush, then season with the garlic powder.
2. Combine the black and the white sesame seeds. Embed them in the tuna steaks, covering the fish all over. Place the tuna into your Air Fry.
3. Cook for 8 minutes at 400°F, turning the fish halfway through.
4. The tuna steaks are ready when they have reached a temperature of 145°F. Serve straightaway.

Nutrition:
- Calories: 343
- Fats: 11 g
- Carbs: 27 g
- Protein: 25 g

Lemon Garlic Shrimp

Preparation Time: 5 minutes
Cooking Time: 10 minutes
Servings: 4
Ingredients:
- 1 medium lemon
- ½ lb. medium shrimp, shelled and deveined
- ½ tsp. OLD BAY® seasoning
- 2 tbsp. unsalted butter, melted

Directions:
1. Grate the lemon rind into a bowl. Cut the lemon in half then juice it in the same bowl. Toss in the shrimp, OLD BAY®, and butter, mixing

everything to make sure the shrimp is completely covered.
2. Transfer to a round baking dish roughly 6 inches wide, then place this dish in your Air Fry Oven.
3. Cook at 400°F for 6 minutes. The shrimp is ready when it becomes a bright pink color.
4. Serve hot, drizzling any leftover sauce over the shrimp.

Nutrition:
- Calories: 374
- Fats: 14 g
- Carbs: 18 g
- Protein: 21 g

Foil Packet Salmon

Preparation Time: 5 minutes
Cooking Time: 10 minutes
Servings: 4
Ingredients:
- 2 (4-oz.) salmon fillets, skinless
- 2 tbsp. unsalted butter, melted
- ½ tsp. garlic powder
- 1 medium lemon
- ½ tsp. dried dill

Directions:
1. Take a sheet of foil and cut into two squares measuring roughly 5"x5". Lay each of the salmon fillets at the center of each piece. Brush both fillets with 1 tbsp. of butter and season with ¼ tsp. of garlic powder.
2. Halve the lemon and grate the skin of one half over the fish. Cut four half-slices of lemon, using two to top each fillet. Season each fillet with ¼ tsp. of dill.
3. Fold the tops and sides of the aluminum foil over the fish to create a kind of packet. Place each one in the fryer.
4. Cook for 12 minutes at 400°F.
5. The salmon is ready when it flakes easily. Serve hot.

Nutrition:
- Calories: 365
- Fats: 16 g
- Carbs: 18 g
- Protein: 23 g

Foil Packet Lobster Tail

Preparation Time: 5 minutes
Cooking Time: 10 minutes
Servings: 4
Ingredients:

- 2 (6-oz.) lobster tail halves
- 2 tbsp. salted butter, melted
- ½ medium lemon, juiced
- ½ tsp. OLD BAY® seasoning
- 1 tsp. dried parsley

Directions:

1. Lay each lobster on a sheet of aluminum foil. Add ½ of the butter and lemon juice over each one, and season with OLD BAY®.
2. Fold down the sides and ends of the foil to seal the lobster. Place each one in the fryer.
3. Cook at 375°F for 12 minutes.
4. Just before serving, top the lobster with dried parsley.

Nutrition:

- Calories: 369
- Fats: 19 g
- Carbs: 25 g
- Protein: 28 g

Avocado Shrimp

Preparation Time: 5 minutes
Cooking Time: 10 minutes
Servings: 4
Ingredients:

- ½ cup onion, chopped
- 2 lb. shrimp
- 1 tbsp. seasoned salt
- 1 avocado
- ½ cup pecans, chopped

Directions:

1. Preheat the fryer to 400°F.
2. Put the chopped onion in the basket of the fryer and spritz with some cooking spray. Let cook for 5 minutes.
3. Add the shrimp and set the timer for a further 5 minutes. Sprinkle with some seasoned salt, then allow to cook for an additional 5 minutes.
4. During these last 5 minutes, halve your avocado and remove the pit. Cube each half, then scoop out the flesh.

5. Take care when removing the shrimp from the Air Fry Oven. Place it on a dish and top with the avocado and the chopped pecans.

Nutrition:

- Calories: 384
- Fats: 24 g
- Carbs: 13 g
- Protein: 39 g

Lemon Butter Scallops

Preparation Time: 1 hour 5 minutes
Cooking Time: 10 minutes
Servings: 4
Ingredients:

- 1 lemon
- 1 lb. scallops
- ½ cup butter
- ¼ cup parsley, chopped

Directions:

1. Juice the lemon into a Ziploc® bag.
2. Wash your scallops, dry them, and season to taste. Put them in the bag with the lemon juice. Refrigerate for 1 hour.
3. Remove the bag from the refrigerator and leave for about 12 minutes, or until it returns to room temperature. Transfer the scallops into a foil pan that is small enough to be placed inside the fryer.
4. Preheat the fryer to 400°F and put the rack inside.
5. Place the foil pan on the rack, and cook for five minutes.
6. In the meantime, melt the butter in a saucepan over medium heat. Zest the lemon over the saucepan, then add in the chopped parsley. Mix well.
7. Be careful when removing the pan from the Air Fry Oven. Transfer the contents to a plate and drizzle with the lemon-butter mixture. Serve hot.

Nutrition:

- Calories: 412
- Fats: 17 g
- Carbs: 18 g
- Protein: 26 g

Cheesy Lemon Halibut

Preparation Time: 5 minutes
Cooking Time: 10 minutes
Servings: 4

Ingredients:
- 1 lb. halibut fillet
- ½ cup butter
- 2 ½ tbsp. mayonnaise
- 2 ½ tbsp. lemon juice
- ¾ cup parmesan cheese, grated
- ½ tsp. Cooking spray

Directions:
1. Preheat your fryer to 375°F.
2. Spritz the halibut fillets with cooking spray and season as desired.
3. Put the halibut in the fryer and cook for 12 minutes.
4. In the meantime, combine the butter, mayonnaise, and lemon juice in a bowl with a hand mixer. Ensure a creamy texture is achieved.
5. Stir in the grated parmesan.
6. When the halibut is ready, open the Air Fry Oven and spread the butter over the fish with a butter knife. Let it cook for a couple more minutes, then serve hot.

Nutrition:
- Calories: 354
- Fats: 21 g
- Carbs: 23 g
- Protein: 19 g

Spicy Mackerel

Preparation Time: 5 minutes
Cooking Time: 10 minutes
Servings: 4
Ingredients:
- 2 mackerel fillets
- 2 tbsp. red pepper flakes
- 2 tsp. garlic, minced
- 1 tsp. lemon juice

Directions:
1. Season the mackerel fillets with the red pepper flakes, minced garlic, and a drizzle of lemon juice. Allow to sit for 5 minutes.
2. Preheat your fryer at 350°F.
3. Cook the mackerel for 5 minutes, before opening the Air Fry Oven to flip the fillets, allow to cook on the other side for another 5 minutes.
4. Plate the fillets, making sure to spoon any remaining juice over them before serving.

Nutrition:
- Calories: 393
- Fats: 12 g
- Carbs: 13 g
- Protein: 35 g

CHAPTER 8: DEHYDRATE

Pineapple Slices

Preparation Time: 10 minutes
Cooking Time: 14 hours
Servings: 12
Ingredients:
- 12 pineapple slices

Directions:
1. Select "Dehydrate" mode.
2. Select "LEVEL 2," then set time for 14 hours and set the temperature to 125ºF.
3. Place the pineapple slices in the air fry basket and place the basket in the Air Fry Oven. Press "Start."

Nutrition:
- Calories: 374
- Fats: 0.9 g
- Carbs: 99 g
- Sugar: 74.5 g
- Protein: 4.1 g

Apple Slices

Preparation Time: 10 minutes
Cooking Time: 8 hours
Servings: 4
Ingredients:
- 2 apple, cored and cut into ⅛-inch thick slices
- 1 tsp. ground cinnamon

Directions:
1. Select "Dehydrate" mode.
2. Select "LEVEL 2," then set time for 8 hours and set the temperature to 145ºF.
3. Place the apple slices in the air fry basket and place the basket in the Air Fry Oven.
4. Sprinkle cinnamon on top of the apple slices.
5. Press "Start."

Nutrition:
- Calories: 60
- Fats: 0.2 g
- Carbs: 16 g
- Sugar: 11.6 g
- Protein: 0.3 g

Pear Slices

Preparation Time: 10 minutes
Cooking Time: 5 hours
Servings: 4
Ingredients:
- 2 pears, cut into ¼ -inch thick slices

Directions:
1. Select "Dehydrate" mode.
2. Select "LEVEL 2," then set time for 5 hours and set the temperature to 160ºF.
3. Place the pear slices in the air fry basket and place the basket in the Air Fry Oven. Press "Start."

Nutrition:
- Calories: 61
- Fats: 0.2 g
- Carbs: 16 g
- Sugar: 10.2 g
- Protein: 0.4 g

Mango Slices

Preparation Time: 10 minutes
Cooking Time: 12 hours
Servings: 4
Ingredients:
- 2 large mangoes, peeled and cut into ¼ -inch thick slices

Directions:
1. Select "Dehydrate" mode.
2. Select "LEVEL 2," then set time for 12 hours and set the temperature to 135ºF.
3. Place the mango slices in the air fry basket and place the basket in the Air Fry Oven. Press "Start."

Nutrition:
- Calories: 102
- Fats: 0.6 g
- Carbs: 25 g
- Sugar: 23 g
- Protein: 1.4 g

Zucchini Slices

Preparation Time: 10 minutes
Cooking Time: 12 hours
Servings: 4
Ingredients:
- 1 zucchini, sliced thinly

Directions:
1. Select "Dehydrate" mode.

1.   Select "LEVEL 2," then set time for 12 hours and set the temperature to 135ºF.

2.   Place the zucchini slices in the air fry basket and place the basket in the Air Fry Oven. Press "Start."

Nutrition:
- Calories: 10
- Fats: 0.1 g
- Carbs: 2.1 g
- Sugar: 0.9 g
- Protein: 0.6 g

Dragon Fruit Slices

Preparation Time: 10 minutes
Cooking Time: 12 hours
Servings: 4
Ingredients:
- 2 dragon fruit, peeled and cut into ¼ -inch thick slices

Directions:
1.   Select "Dehydrate" mode.

2.   Select "LEVEL 2," then set time for 12 hours and set the temperature to 115ºF.

3.   Place the dragon fruit slices in the air fry basket and place the basket in the Air Fry Oven. Press "Start."

Nutrition:
- Calories: 25
- Carbs: 6 g
- Sugar: 6 g

Broccoli Florets

Preparation Time: 10 minutes
Cooking Time: 12 hours
Servings: 6
Ingredients:
- 1 lb. broccoli florets
- Pepper
- Salt

Directions:
1.   Select "Dehydrate" mode.

2.   Select "LEVEL 2," then set time for 12 hours and set the temperature to 115ºF.

3.   Place the broccoli florets in the air fry basket and place the basket in the Air Fry Oven. Press "Start."

Nutrition:
- Calories: 25

- Fats: 0.3 g
- Carbs: 5 g
- Sugar: 1.3 g
- Protein: 2.1 g

Avocado Slices

Preparation Time: 10 minutes
Cooking Time: 10 hours
Servings: 4
Ingredients:
- 4 avocados, halved and pitted

Directions:
1.   Select "Dehydrate" mode.

2.   Select "LEVEL 2," then set time for 10 hours and set the temperature to 160ºF.

3.   Place the avocado slices in the air fry basket and place the basket in the Air Fry Oven. Press "Start."

Nutrition:
- Calories: 415
- Fats: 39 g
- Carbs: 17.5 g
- Sugar: 1.1 g
- Protein: 3.9 g

Sweet Potato Chips

Preparation Time: 10 minutes
Cooking Time: 12 hours
Servings: 2
Ingredients:
- 2 sweet potatoes, peel and sliced thinly
- 1 tsp. olive oil
- ⅛ tsp. cinnamon
- Salt

Directions:
1.   Add the sweet potato slices in a bowl. Add the cinnamon, oil, and salt and toss well.

2.   Select "Dehydrate" mode.

3.   Select "LEVEL 2," then set time for 12 hours and set the temperature to 125ºF.

4.   Place the sweet potato slices in the air fry basket and place the basket in the Air Fry Oven. Press "Start."

Nutrition:
- Calories: 195
- Fats: 2 g
- Carbs: 41 g
- Sugar: 0.8 g

- Protein: 2.3 g

Kiwi Chips

Preparation Time: 5 minutes

Cooking Time: 10 hours

Servings: 4

Ingredients:

- 6 kiwis, peeled & cut into ¼ -inch thick slices

Directions:

1. Select "Dehydrate" mode.

2. Select "LEVEL 2,"then set time for 10 hours and set the temperature to 135ºF.

3. Place kiwi slices in the air fry basket and place the basket in the Air Fry Oven. Press "Start."

Nutrition:

- Calories: 71
- Fats: 0.6 g
- Carbs: 16 g
- Sugar: 10.3 g
- Protein: 1.3 g

CHAPTER 9: DESSERTS

Perfect Cinnamon Toast

Preparation Time: 10 minutes
Cooking Time: 5 minutes
Servings: 6
Ingredients:

- 2 tsp. pepper
- 1 ½ tsp. cinnamon
- ½ cup sweetener of choice
- 1 cup coconut oil
- 12 slices whole wheat bread

Directions:

1. Melt the coconut oil and mix it with the sweetener until dissolved. Mix in the remaining ingredients except bread until incorporated.
2. Spread mixture onto the bread slices, covering all the areas.
3. Pour the coated bread pieces into the oven rack/basket. Place the rack on the middle shelf of the Air Fry Oven. Set temperature to 400°F, and set the time to 5 minutes.
4. Remove and cut diagonally. Enjoy!

Nutrition:

- Calories: 124
- Fats: 2 g
- Carbs: 5 g

Angel Food Cake

Preparation Time: 5 minutes
Cooking Time: 30 minutes
Servings: 12
Ingredients:

- ¼ cup butter, melted
- 1 cup powdered erythritol
- 1 tsp. strawberry extract
- 12 egg whites
- 2 tsp. cream of tartar

Directions:

1. Preheat the Air Fry Oven for 5 minutes.
2. Blend the cream of tartar and the egg whites.
3. Use a hand mixer and whisk until white and fluffy.
4. Add the rest of the ingredients except for the butter and whisk for another minute.
5. Pour into a baking dish.
6. Place in the air fry basket and cook for 30 minutes at 400°F or if a toothpick inserted in the middle comes out clean.
7. Drizzle with the melted butter once cooled.

Nutrition:

- Calories: 65
- Protein: 3.1 g
- Fats: 5 g
- Carbs: 6.2 g

Apple Dumplings

Preparation Time: 10 minutes
Cooking Time: 25 minutes
Servings: 4
Ingredients:

- 2 tbsp. melted coconut oil
- 2 puff pastry sheets
- 1 tbsp. brown sugar
- 2 tbsp. raisins
- 2 small apples of choice

Directions:

1. Preheat the Air Fry Oven to 356ºF.
2. Core and peel the apples and mix with the raisins and sugar.
3. Place a bit of the apple mixture into the puff pastry sheets and brush the sides with the melted coconut oil.
4. Place into the Air Fry Oven. Cook for 25 minutes, turning halfway through. They will be golden when done.

Nutrition:

- Calories: 367
- Protein: 2 g
- Fats: 7 g
- Carbs: 10 g

Chocolate Donuts

Preparation Time: 5 minutes
Cooking Time: 20 minutes
Servings: 8–10
Ingredients:

- (8-oz.) can Jumbo® biscuits
- 1 tbsp Cooking oil

- 2 tbsp Chocolate sauce, such as Betty Crocker™

Directions:

1. Form 8 donuts out of the dough and place them on a flat worksurface. Use a small circle cookie cutter or a biscuit cutter to cut a hole in the center of each donut. You can also cut the holes using a knife.
2. Grease the basket with cooking oil.
3. Place 4 donuts in the Air Fry Oven. Do not stack. Spray with cooking oil. Cook for 4 minutes.
4. Open the Air Fry Oven and flip the donuts. Cook for an additional 4 minutes.
5. Remove the cooked donuts from the Air Fry Oven, then repeat for the remaining 4 donuts.
6. Drizzle chocolate sauce over the donuts and enjoy while warm.

Nutrition:

- Calories: 181
- Protein: 3 g
- Fats: 98 g
- Carbs: 42 g

Apple Hand Pies

Preparation Time: 5 minutes
Cooking Time: 8 minutes
Servings: 6
Ingredients:

- 15 oz. apple pie filling, no-sugar-added
- 1 store-bought pie crust

Directions:

1. Lay out the pie crust and slice them into equal-sized squares.
2. Place 2 tbsp. of apple pie filling into each square and seal the crust with a fork.
3. Place the Rack on the middle shelf of the Air Fry Oven. Set temperature to 390°F, and set the time to 8 minutes, or until golden in color.

Nutrition:

- Calories: 278
- Protein: 5 g
- Fats: 10 g
- Carbs: 17 g

Sweet Cream Cheese Wontons

Preparation Time: 5 minutes
Cooking Time: 5 minutes
Servings: 16

Ingredients:

- 1 egg with a little water
- 2 Wonton wrappers
- ½ cup powdered erythritol
- 8 oz. softened cream cheese
- 1 tbsp Olive oil

Directions:

1. Mix the sweetener and the cream cheese together.
2. Lay out 4 wontons at a time and cover with a dish towel to prevent them from drying out.
3. Place ½ of a tsp. of cream cheese mixture into each wrapper.
4. Dip your finger into the egg-water mixture and fold it diagonally to form a triangle. Seal the edges well.
5. Repeat with the remaining ingredients.
6. Place filled wontons into the Air Fry Oven and cook 5 minutes at 400°F, shaking halfway through cooking.

Nutrition:

- Calories: 303
- Protein: 0.5 g
- Fats: 3 g
- Carbs: 3 g

French Toast Bites

Preparation Time: 5 minutes
Cooking Time: 15 minutes
Servings: 8
Ingredients:

- 3 tbsp Almond milk
- 1 tbsp Cinnamon sugar to taste
- ⅓ cup sweetener
- 3 eggs
- 4 pieces wheat bread

Directions:

1. Preheat the Air Fry Oven to 360°F.
2. Whisk the eggs and thin out with almond milk.
3. Mix ⅓ cup of sweetener with lots of cinnamon.
4. Tear the bread in half, ball up pieces and press together to form a ball.
5. Soak the bread balls in the egg mixture, and then into cinnamon sugar, making sure to thoroughly coat.

6.   Place the coated bread balls into the Air Fry Oven and bake for 15 minutes.

Nutrition:

- Calories: 289
- Fats: 11 g
- Carbs: 17 g

Cinnamon Sugar Roasted Chickpeas

Preparation Time: 5 minutes
Cooking Time: 10 minutes
Servings: 2
Ingredients:

- 1 tbsp. sweetener
- 1 tbsp. cinnamon
- 1 cup chickpeas

Directions:

1.   Preheat th Air Fry Oven to 390ºF.
2.   Rinse and drain the chickpeas.
3.   Mix all the ingredients together and add to the Air Fry Oven.
4.   Pour into the oven rack/basket. Place the rack on the middle shelf of the Air Fry Oven. Set temperature to 390°F, and set time to 10 minutes.

Nutrition:

- Calories: 111
- Protein: 16 g
- Fats: 19 g
- Carbs: 18 g

Brownie Muffins

Preparation Time: 10 minutes
Cooking Time: 10 minutes
Servings: 12
Ingredients:

- 1 package Betty Crocker™ Fudge Brownie Mix
- ¼ cup walnuts, chopped
- 1 egg
- ⅓ cup vegetable oil
- 2 tsp. water

Directions:

1.   Grease a 12-cavity muffin pan and set it aside.
2.   In a bowl, put all the ingredients together.
3.   Place the mixture into the prepared muffin pan.

4.   Press the "Power" of the Air Fry Oven and turn the dial to select the "Air Fry" mode.
5.   Press the "Time" button and again turn the dial to set the cooking time to 10 minutes.
6.   Now push the "Temp" button and rotate the dial to set the temperature at 300ºF.
7.   Press the "Start/Pause" button to start.
8.   Open the unit when it has reached the temperature, when it beeps.
9.   Arrange the muffin pan in the air fry basket and insert it in the oven.
10.   Place the muffin pan onto a wire rack to cool for about 10 minutes.
11.   Carefully, invert the muffins onto the wire rack to completely cool before serving.

Nutrition:

- Calories: 168
- Protein: 2 g
- Fats: 8.9 g
- Carbs: 20.8 g

Chocolate Mug Cake

Preparation Time: 15 minutes
Cooking Time: 13 minutes
Servings: 1
Ingredients:

- ¼ cup self-rising flour
- 5 tbsp. caster sugar
- 1 tbsp. cocoa powder
- 3 tbsp. coconut oil
- 3 tbsp. whole milk

Directions:

1.   In a shallow mug, add all the ingredients and mix until well combined.
2.   Press the "Power" of the Air Fry Oven and turn the dial to select the "Air Fry" mode.
3.   Press the "Time" button and again turn the dial to set the cooking time to 13 minutes.
4.   Now push the "Temp" button and rotate the dial to set the temperature at 392ºF.
5.   Press the "Start/Pause" button to start.
6.   Open the unit when it has reached the temperature, when it beeps.
7.   Arrange the mug in the air fry basket and insert it in the Air Fry Oven.
8.   Place the mug onto a wire rack to cool slightly before serving.

Nutrition:

- Calories: 729
- Protein: 5.7 g
- Fats: 43.3 g
- Carbs: 88.8 g

Grilled Peaches

Preparation Time: 10 minutes
Cooking Time: 10 minutes
Servings: 2
Ingredients:

- 2 peaches, cut into wedges and remove pits
- ¼ cup butter, diced into pieces
- ¼ cup brown sugar
- ¼ cup Graham Cracker® crumbs

Directions:

1. Arrange the peach wedges on air fry oven rack and air-fry at 350ºF for 5 minutes.
2. In a bowl, add the butter, Graham Cracker® crumbs, and brown sugar and mix well.
3. Place the pecans skin-side down.
4. Spoon the butter mixture over top of the peaches and air-fry for 5 minutes more.
5. Top with the whipped cream and serve.

Nutrition:

- Calories: 378
- Protein: 2.3 g
- Fats: 24.4 g
- Carbs: 40.5 g

Simple & Delicious Spiced Apples

Preparation Time: 10 minutes
Cooking Time: 10 minutes
Servings: 4
Ingredients:

- 4 apples, sliced
- 1 tsp. apple pie spice
- 2 tbsp. sugar
- 2 tbsp. ghee, melted
- 2 lb. Ice cream

Directions:

1. Add the apple slices into the mixing bowl.
2. Add the remaining ingredients on top of the apple slices and toss until well coated.
3. Transfer apple slices on the ninja foodi digital air fryer oven pan and air-fry at 350ºF for 10 minutes.

4. Top with the ice cream and serve.

Nutrition:

- Calories: 196
- Protein: 0.6 g
- Fats: 6.8 g
- Carbs: 37.1 g

Tangy Mango Slices

Preparation Time: 10 minutes
Cooking Time: 12 hours
Servings: 6
Ingredients:

- 4 mangoes, peeled and cut into ¼-inch slices
- ¼ cup fresh lemon juice
- 1 tbsp. honey

Directions:

1. In a big bowl, combine together the honey and lemon juice and set aside.
2. Add the mango slices in the lemon-honey mixture and coat them well.
3. Arrange the mango slices on the ninja foodi digital air fryer rack and dehydrate them at 135ºF for 12 hours.

Nutrition:

- Calories: 147
- Protein: 1.9 g
- Fats: 0.9 g
- Carbs: 36.7 g

Dried Raspberries

Preparation Time: 10 minutes
Cooking Time: 15 hours
Servings: 4
Ingredients:

- 4 cups raspberries, washed and dried
- ¼ cup fresh lemon juice

Directions:

1. Add the raspberries and lemon juice in a bowl and toss well.
2. Arrange the raspberries on the ninja foodi digital air fryer oven tray and dehydrate them at 135ºF for 12–15 hours.
3. Store in an air-tight container.

Nutrition:

- Calories: 68
- Protein: 1.6 g

- Fats: 0.9 g
- Carbs: 15 g

Sweet Peach Wedges

Preparation Time: 10 minutes
Cooking Time: 8 hours
Servings: 4
Ingredients:
- 3 peaches, cut and remove pits and sliced
- ½ cup fresh lemon juice

Directions:
1. Add the lemon juice and the peach slices into the bowl and toss well.
2. Arrange the peach slices on the ninja foodi digital air fryer oven rack and dehydrate them at 135ºF for 6–8 hours.
3. Serve and enjoy.

Nutrition:
- Calories: 52
- Protein: 1.3 g
- Fats: 0.5 g
- Carbs: 11.1 g

Air Fryer Oreo Cookies

Preparation Time: 5 minutes
Cooking Time: 5 minutes
Servings: 9
Ingredients:
- ½ cup pancake mix:
- ½ cup water:
- Cooking spray
- 9 chocolate sandwich cookies: (e.g. Oreo®)
- 1 tbsp. (or to taste) confectioners' sugar

Directions:
1. Blend the pancake mix with the water until well mixed.
2. Line the parchment paper on the air fry basket. Spray non-stick cooking spray on the parchment paper. Dip each cookie in the pancake mix and place them in the basket. Make sure they do not touch; if possible, cook in batches.
3. Preheat the Air Fry Oven to 400°F. Cook for 4–5 minutes; flip until golden brown, 2–3 more minutes. Sprinkle the confectioners' sugar over the cookies and serve.

Nutrition:
- Calories: 77

- Protein: 1.2 g
- Fats: 2.1 g
- Carbs: 13.7 g

Air Fried Butter Cake

Preparation Time: 10 minutes
Cooking Time: 15 minutes
Servings: 4
Ingredients:
- 7 tbsp. butter, at ambient temperature
- ¼ cup white sugar, plus 2 tbsp.
- 1 ⅔ cups all-purpose flour
- 1 pinch salt, or to taste
- 6 tbsp. milk

Directions:
1. Preheat the Air Fry Oven to 350ºF. Spray the cooking spray on a tiny fluted tube pan.
2. Take a large bowl and add ¼ cup butter and 2 tbsp. of sugar in it.
3. Take an electric mixer to beat the sugar and butter until smooth and fluffy. Stir in the salt and flour. Stir in the milk and thoroughly combine the batter. Transfer the batter to the prepared saucepan; use a spoon back to level the surface.
4. Place the pan inside the air fry basket. Set the timer within 15 minutes. Bake the batter until a toothpick comes out clean when inserted into the cake.
5. Turn the cake out of the saucepan and allow it to cool for about 5 minutes.

Nutrition:
- Calories: 470
- Protein: 7.9 g
- Fats: 22.4 g
- Carbs: 59.7 g

Air Fryer S'mores

Preparation Time: 5 minutes
Cooking Time: 3 minutes
Servings: 4
Ingredients:
- 4 Graham Crackers®, each half split to make 2 squares, for a total of 8 squares
- 8 squares chocolate bar Hershey's® , broken into squares
- 4 marshmallows

Directions:

1. Take deliberate steps. Air-fryers use hot air for cooking food. Marshmallows are light and fluffy, and this should keep the marshmallows from flying around the basket if you follow these steps.

2. Put 4 squares of Graham Crackers® on a basket of the air fryer.

3. Place 2 squares of chocolate bars on each cracker.

4. Place the basket back into the Air Fry Oven and fry at 390°F for 1 minute. It is barely long enough for the chocolate to melt. Remove basket from air fryer.

5. Top with a marshmallow over each cracker. Throw the marshmallow down a little bit into the melted chocolate. This will help in making the marshmallow stay over the chocolate.

6. Put the basket back into the Air Fry Oven and fry at 390°F for 2 minutes. (The marshmallows should be puffed up and browned at the tops).

7. Using tongs to carefully remove each cracker from the air fry basket and place it on a platter. Top each marshmallow with another square of Graham Crackers®.

8. Enjoy it right away!

Nutrition:
- Calories: 200
- Protein: 2.6 g
- Fats: 3.1 g
- Carbs: 15.7 g

Peanut Butter Cookies

Preparation Time: 2 minutes
Cooking Time: 5 minutes
Servings: 10
Ingredients:
- 1 cup peanut butter
- 1 cup sugar
- 1 egg

Directions:
1. Blend all of the ingredients with a hand mixer.

2. Spray the air fry basket with canola oil. (Alternatively, parchment paper can also be used, but it will take longer to cook your cookies)

3. Set the Air Fry Oven temperature to 350ºF.

4. Place rounded dough balls onto air fryer trays. Press down softly with the back of a fork.

5. Place air fry basket in your Air Fry Oven in the middle shelf. Cook for 5 minutes.

6. Serve the cookies with milk.

Nutrition:
- Calories: 236
- Protein: 6 g
- Fats: 13 g
- Carbs: 26 g

Sweet Pear Stew

Preparation Time: 10 minutes
Cooking Time: 15 minutes
Servings: 4
Ingredients:
- 4 pears, cored and cut into wedges
- 1 tsp. vanilla
- ¼ cup apple juice
- 2 cups grapes, halved

Directions:
1. Put all of the ingredients in the ninja foodi digital air fryer oven and stir well.

2. Close the ninja foodi digital air fryer oven and cook on high for 15 minutes.

3. As soon as the cooking is done, let it release pressure naturally for 10 minutes, then release the remaining pressure using "Quick Release." Remove the lid.

4. Stir and serve.

Nutrition:
- Calories: 162
- Protein: 1.1 g
- Fats: 0.5 g
- Carbs: 41.6 g

Vanilla Apple Compote

Preparation Time: 10 minutes
Cooking Time: 15 minutes
Servings: 6
Ingredients:
- 3 cups apples, cored and cubed
- 1 tsp. vanilla
- ¾ cup coconut sugar
- 1 cup water
- 2 tbsp. fresh lime juice

Directions:
1. Put all of the ingredients in the instnt pot and stir well.

2. Close the ninja foodi digital air fryer oven and cook on high for 15 minutes.

3. As soon as the cooking is done, let it release pressure naturally for 10 minutes, then release the remaining pressure using "Quick Release." Remove the lid.

4. Stir and serve.

Nutrition:
- Calories: 76
- Protein: 0.5 g
- Fats: 0.2 g
- Carbs: 19.1 g

Apple Dates Mix

Preparation Time: 10 minutes
Cooking Time: 15 minutes
Servings: 4
Ingredients:
- 4 apples, cored and cut into chunks
- 1 tsp. vanilla
- 1 tsp. cinnamon
- ½ cup dates, pitted
- 1 ½ cups apple juice

Directions:
1. Put all of the ingredients in the ninja foodi digital air fryer oven and stir well.

2. Close the ninja foodi digital air fryer oven and cook on high for 15 minutes.

3. As soon as the cooking is done, let release pressure naturally for 10 minutes, then release the remaining pressure using "Quick Release." Remove the lid.

4. Stir and serve.

Nutrition:
- Calories: 226
- Protein: 1.3 g
- Fats: 0.6 g
- Carbs: 58.6 g

Chocolate Rice

Preparation Time: 10 minutes
Cooking Time: 20 minutes
Servings: 4
Ingredients:
- 1 cup rice
- 1 tbsp. cocoa powder
- 2 tbsp. maple syrup

- 2 cups almond milk

Directions:
1. Put all of the ingredients in the ninja foodi digital air fryer oven and stir well.

2. Close the ninja foodi digital air fryer oven and cook on high for 20 minutes.

3. As soon as the cooking is done, let it cool naturally for 10 minutes, then release the remaining pressure using "Quick Release." Remove the lid.

4. Stir and serve.

Nutrition:
- Calories: 474
- Protein: 6.3 g
- Fats: 29.1 g
- Carbs: 51.1 g

Raisins Cinnamon Peaches

Preparation Time: 10 minutes
Cooking Time: 15 minutes
Servings: 4
Ingredients:
- 4 peaches, cored and cut into chunks
- 1 tsp. vanilla
- 1 tsp. cinnamon
- ½ cup raisins
- 1 cup water

Directions:
1. Put all of the ingredients in the ninja foodi digital air fryer oven and stir well.

2. Close the ninja foodi digital air fryer oven and cook on high for 15 minutes.

3. As soon as the cooking is done, let it release pressure naturally for 10 minutes, then release the remaining pressure using "Quick Release." Remove the lid.

4. Stir and serve.

Nutrition:
- Calories: 118
- Protein: 2 g
- Fats: 0.5 g
- Carbs: 29 g

Lemon Pear Compote

Preparation Time: 10 minutes
Cooking Time: 15 minutes
Servings: 6
Ingredients:

- 3 cups pears, cored and cut into chunks
- 1 tsp. vanilla
- 1 tsp. liquid stevia
- 1 tbsp. lemon zest, grated
- 2 tbsp. lemon juice

Directions:

1. Put all of the ingredients in the ninja foodi digital air fryer oven and stir well.
2. Close the ninja foodi digital air fryer oven and cook on high for 15 minutes.
3. As soon as the cooking is done, let it release pressure naturally for 10 minutes, then release the remaining pressure using "Quick Release." Remove the lid.
4. Stir and serve.

Nutrition:

- Calories: 50
- Protein: 0.4 g
- Fats: 0.2 g
- Carbs: 12.7 g

Strawberry Stew

Preparation Time: 10 minutes
Cooking Time: 15 minutes
Servings: 4
Ingredients:

- 12 oz. fresh strawberries, sliced
- 1 tsp. vanilla
- 1 ½ cups water
- 1 tsp. liquid stevia
- 2 tbsp. lime juice

Directions:

1. Put all of the ingredients in the ninja foodi digital air fryer oven and stir well.
2. Close the ninja foodi digital air fryer oven and cook on high for 15 minutes.
3. As soon as the cooking is done, let it release pressure naturally for 10 minutes, then release the remaining pressure using "Quick Release." Remove the lid.
4. Stir and serve.

Nutrition:

- Calories: 36
- Protein: 0.7 g
- Fats: 0.3 g
- Carbs: 8.5 g

Walnut Apple Pear Mix

Preparation Time: 10 minutes
Cooking Time: 10 minutes
Servings: 4
Ingredients:

- 2 apples, cored and cut into wedges
- ½ tsp. vanilla
- 1 cup apple juice
- 2 tbsp. walnuts, chopped
- 2 apples, cored and cut into wedges

Directions:

1. Put all of the ingredients in the ninja foodi digital air fryer oven and stir well.
2. Close the ninja foodi digital air fryer oven and cook on high for 10 minutes.
3. As soon as the cooking is done, let it release pressure naturally for 10 minutes, then release the remaining pressure using "Quick Release." Remove the lid.
4. Serve and enjoy.

Nutrition:

- Calories: 132
- Protein: 1.3 g
- Fats: 2.6 g
- Carbs: 28.3 g

Cinnamon Pear Jam

Preparation Time: 10 minutes
Cooking Time: 4 minutes
Servings: 12
Ingredients:

- 8 pears, cored and cut into quarters
- 1 tsp. cinnamon
- ¼ cup apple juice
- 2 apples, peeled, cored and diced

Directions:

1. Put all of the ingredients in the ninja foodi digital air fryer oven and stir well.
2. Close the ninja foodi digital air fryer oven and cook on high for 4 minutes.
3. As soon as the cooking is done, let it release pressure naturally. Remove the lid.
4. Blend the pear apple mixture using an immersion blender until smooth.
5. Serve and enjoy.

Nutrition:

- Calories: 103

- Protein: 0.6 g
- Fats: 0.3 g
- Carbs: 27.1 g

Pear Sauce

Preparation Time: 10 minutes
Cooking Time: 15 minutes
Servings: 6
Ingredients:
- 10 pears, sliced
- 1 cup apple juice
- 1 ½ tsp. cinnamon
- ¼ tsp. nutmeg

Directions:
1. Put all of the ingredients in the ninja foodi digital air fryer oven and stir well.
2. Close the ninja foodi digital air fryer oven and cook on high for 15 minutes.
3. Once done, allow to release pressure naturally for 10 minutes, then release the remaining using "Quick Release." Remove the lid.
4. Blend the pear mixture using an immersion blender until smooth.
5. Serve and enjoy.

Nutrition:
- Calories: 222
- Protein: 1.3 g
- Fats: 0.6 g
- Carbs: 58.2 g

Sweet Peach Jam

Preparation Time: 10 minutes
Cooking Time: 16 minutes
Servings: 20
Ingredients:
- 1 ½ lb. fresh peaches, pitted and chopped
- ½ tbsp. vanilla
- ¼ cup maple syrup

Directions:
1. Put all of the ingredients in the ninja foodi digital air fryer oven and stir well.
2. Close the ninja foodi digital air fryer oven and cook on high for 1 minute.
3. Once done, allow to release pressure naturally. Remove the lid.
4. Set pot on "Sauté" mode and cook for 15 minutes, or until the jam is thickened.

5. Pour into the container and store it in the fridge.

Nutrition:
- Calories: 16
- Protein: 0.1 g
- Carbs: 3.7 g

Warm Peach Compote

Preparation Time: 10 minutes
Cooking Time: 1 minute
Servings: 4
Ingredients:
- 4 peaches, peeled and chopped
- 1 tbsp. water
- ½ tbsp. cornstarch
- 1 tsp. vanilla

Directions:
1. Add the water, vanilla, and peaches into the ninja foodi digital air fryer oven.
2. Close the ninja foodi digital air fryer oven and cook on high for 1 minute.
3. Once done, allow to release pressure naturally. Remove the lid.
4. In a small bowl, whisk together 1 tbsp. of water and the cornstarch and pour into the pot and stir well.
5. Serve and enjoy.

Nutrition:
- Calories: 66
- Protein: 1.4 g
- Fats: 0.4 g
- Carbs: 15 g

Spiced Pear Sauce

Preparation Time: 10 minutes
Cooking Time: 6 hours
Servings: 12
Ingredients:
- 8 pears, cored and diced
- ½ tsp. ground cinnamon
- ¼ tsp. ground nutmeg
- ¼ tsp. ground cardamom
- 1 cup water

Directions:
1. Put all of the ingredients in the ninja foodi digital air fryer oven and stir well.

2.   Close the ninja foodi digital air fryer oven with its lid and select "Slow Cook" mode and cook on low for 6 hours.

3.   Mash the sauce using a potato masher.

4.   Pour into the container and store.

Nutrition:

- Calories: 81
- Protein: 0.5 g
- Fats: 0.2 g
- Carbs: 21.4 g

Honey Fruit Compote

Preparation Time: 10 minutes

Cooking Time: 3 minutes

Servings: 4

Ingredients:

- ⅓ cup honey
- 1 ½ cups blueberries
- 1 ½ cups raspberries

Directions:

1.   Put all of the ingredients in the ninja foodi digital air fryer oven and stir well.

2.   Close the ninja foodi digital air fryer oven with lid and cook on high for 3 minutes.

3.   Once done, allow to release pressure naturally. Remove the lid.

4.   Serve and enjoy.

Nutrition:

- Calories: 141
- Protein: 1 g
- Fats: 0.5 g
- Carbs: 36.7 g

APPENDIX : RECIPES INDEX

CPSIA information can be obtained
at www.ICGtesting.com
Printed in the USA
BVHW022140200723
667596BV00004B/86